SPENCER AND CHRISTINA KROLL

The Ozempic Diet

First published by Deuterium Press 2023

First edition

This book was professionally typeset on Reedsy.
Find out more at reedsy.com

Contents

Preface

In the intricate world of metabolic medicine, where the dance of molecules determines our health and well-being, I've had the privilege of wearing two intertwined hats: that of a Board Certified Lipid Specialist and a Medical Doctor. The confluence of these roles has provided me with a unique vantage point, from which I've discerned not only the biochemical nuances but also the very tangible, day-to-day struggles and triumphs of my patients.

Ozempic, a name that has become increasingly familiar in the realms of diabetes and weight management, represents a beacon of hope for many. However, like every medication, its potency is intertwined with the lifestyle choices that accompany it. And among those choices, the act of eating—so basic yet so complex—stands out.

This book is not just about a medication. It's about harmonizing the power of Ozempic with the ancient art of nourishment. It's about understanding the symphony of hormones, nutrients, and metabolic processes, and ensuring each note plays to its potential. Through these pages, I aim to provide you with a compass—a guide to eating right while on Ozempic, based on both scientific evidence and clinical experience.

Join me on this journey as we delve into the science, bust myths, and explore the delightful art of crafting meals that not only satisfy your taste buds but also synergize with Ozempic to usher you towards optimal health.

Spencer Kroll MD PhD, Fellow of the National Lipid Association

As a certified clinical nutritionist, I have had the privilege of witnessing countless individuals on their journey to better health. Ozempic and similar medications have shown remarkable potential in helping individuals shed excess pounds and maintain healthy blood sugar levels. However, as with any medical intervention, success often hinges not only on the medication itself but also on the choices individuals make regarding their diet, lifestyle, and their relationship with food.

In this comprehensive guide, I aim to provide Ozempic users and those considering this medication with valuable insights into crafting a diet plan that optimizes their weight loss and minimizes potential side effects. We will explore a myriad of strategies to help you develop a healthier relationship with food, cultivate mindful eating habits, and transform your approach to nutrition. Moreover, we will delve into the science behind Ozempic and its role in blood sugar control, elucidating how dietary choices can complement its effects and contribute to your overall well-being.

Throughout this book, my goal is to empower you with knowledge, practical advice, and evidence-based strategies to make informed decisions about your dietary choices. Whether you're beginning your Ozempic journey or seeking ways to enhance your existing regimen, this guide will serve as a trusted companion on your path to better health, weight management, and improved quality of life. Together, we will explore the symbiotic relationship between nutrition and Ozempic, unlocking the potential for transformative change.

Christina Kroll, Certified Clinical Nutritionist

I

Introduction

1

The Promise Of Weight Loss

Within the successes of contemporary medicine, where numerous advancements have revolutionized healthcare, one innovation has brilliantly stood out. It isn't a magical cure or a solution for every illness, but a product of rigorous science, unwavering dedication, that emerged from a continuous quest to better human lives. This groundbreaking creation is called Ozempic®, set to be a ray of hope for millions fighting the unyielding challenge of diabetes and obesity.

Diabetes, a word that echoes with the weight of its consequences, has been a formidable adversary in the realm of chronic diseases for generations. Its relentless advance has affected the lives of individuals and families worldwide, leaving no corner of the globe untouched. The need for an effective solution, one that not only managed blood sugar levels but also addressed a pressing issue that often accompanies diabetes - weight gain - was a shared dream among both patients and healthcare providers.

Enter Ozempic, a medication that would soon change the course of diabetic care and inspire a renewed sense of optimism. This remarkable medication, the result of tireless research and innovation, was the answer to a long-standing quest for a more effective treatment. But what made Ozempic so extraordinary? It is its remarkable ability to do more than just manage diabetes; it has the power to help individuals shed those stubborn pounds, ushering in a new era of hope and health.

In the pages that follow, we embark on a journey to uncover the story of Ozempic, from its inception in the laboratories of pharmaceutical pioneers to its rise as a game-changer in diabetes management. We will explore the science behind this remarkable medication, hear the stories of those whose lives have been transformed by it, and delve into the broader implications of its arrival on the healthcare stage.

With the enormous popularity of Ozempic, people have come to ask, "What are the best eating guidelines while I am taking this drug?". "Can I eat anything I want?". "What will happen when I stop the medication?" This book will answer these questions and provide Ozempic users with a framework for how to live with this exciting and powerful blockbuster drug.

Novo Nordisk, the pharmaceutical company responsible for producing Ozempic, also offers another medication called Wegovy®, specifically designed and marketed for the treatment of obesity-related weight loss. The information in this book can be used interchangeably in reference to Ozempic and Wegovy, since they share identical ingredients, albeit with varying concentrations.

The story of Ozempic is about the power of human ingenuity and determination to confront one of the greatest health challenges of our time. It's about the individuals who saw a need and worked tirelessly to fill it, the patients who found renewed hope in their battle against diabetes, and the healthcare professionals who witnessed a transformation in their approach to treatment.

Join us as we embark on this journey through the world of Ozempic—a beacon of hope in the fight against diabetes and a promising solution for those seeking not only to control their blood sugar levels but to reclaim their lives and rediscover the joys of health, vitality, and a brighter future.

In the endless pursuit of effective weight loss solutions, the annals of medical history are littered with promises unfulfilled and dreams dashed. For centuries, humans have yearned for a magic bullet to shed excess pounds effortlessly, but the path to this elusive goal has been fraught with challenges and disappointments. In this chapter, we delve into the long and storied history of the search for weight loss drugs, marked by a litany of failures and a determination to overcome them.

The human fascination with weight loss dates back millennia. From ancient Egypt to Greece and beyond, historical records reveal a penchant for concoctions and practices intended to melt away fat. Early remedies often relied on ingredients like vinegar, herbs, and minerals, sometimes coupled with unusual practices like bloodletting and fasting. While some methods may have yielded temporary results, they were far from sustainable or safe.

The mid-20th century saw the emergence of a new player in the weight loss game: amphetamines. These stimulant drugs, known for their appetite-suppressing effects, promised a quick fix to excess weight. In the 1950s and 1960s, amphetamines like Dexedrine and Preludin gained popularity. They did indeed lead to rapid weight loss but at a steep cost. Users experienced a range of side effects, including addiction, heart problems, and psychiatric issues.

The 1990s brought another wave of excitement with the combination of fenfluramine and phentermine, known as Fen-Phen. This duo seemed like a breakthrough, offering effective appetite control with fewer side effects. It gained widespread popularity and was prescribed to millions. However, the party was short-lived. Reports began to surface of serious heart and lung complications, leading to Fen-Phen's eventual withdrawal from the market in the late 1990s. The episode served as a stark reminder of the risks inherent in weight loss drugs.

Orlistat, a medication that inhibits the absorption of dietary fats, entered the scene in the late 1990s under the brand name Xenical and later as an over-the-counter option, Alli. It offered a different approach to weight loss, focusing on fat reduction rather than appetite suppression. While it did prove effective in aiding weight loss, its side effects, which included gastrointestinal distress, limited its appeal to many.

More recently, Belviq and Qsymia emerged as potential weight loss medi-cations. Belviq targeted serotonin receptors to reduce appetite, while Qsymia combined phentermine with topiramate, an anti-seizure medication. These drugs were approved by the FDA, raising hopes once again. However, they faced challenges, including concerns about safety and efficacy, leading to the eventual withdrawal of Belviq from the market in 2020.

The history of weight loss drugs is a testament to the complexity of obesity and the challenges of finding safe and effective solutions. Researchers explored novel approaches, including hormonal therapies and drugs that might work on newly discovered metabolic pathways involved in eating and satiety. The failures of the past did not deter the relentless quest for a medication that could help people achieve lasting and healthy weight loss. And from recent research came several steps that led to the discovery of Semaglutide, marketed as Ozempic.

In the chapters ahead, we will examine the latest breakthroughs in this ongoing narrative - the rise of Ozempic as a potential solution for weight loss in individuals with diabetes and obesity. While history has taught us to approach such innovations with cautious optimism, it is within these stories of past failures that we find the resilience of science and the unwavering commitment to improving the lives of those grappling with obesity and its myriad challenges.

As the buzz surrounding Ozempic has grown, so have questions and skepticism. Is this medication truly a game-changer in the world of diabetes treatment, or is it merely another over-hyped promise destined to fade into the annals of medical history? We will delve deep into the heart of this critical inquiry, seeking to distinguish between the hype and the reality that surrounds Ozempic.

One of the most striking claims associated with Ozempic was its potential for more weight loss than any prior treatment, fad, diet or supplement. For individuals with diabetes, this was a particularly tantalizing prospect. The burden of excess weight often compounded the challenges of managing blood sugar levels. So, when reports emerged of patients shedding pounds while on Ozempic, it ignited hope across the diabetes community.

The reality, as studies and clinical trials would later confirm, was indeed impressive. Ozempic works not only regulating blood sugar but also by curbing appetite and promoting a sense of fullness. This dual mechanism of action leads to weight loss in many patients. However, the extent of weight loss varies from person to person, and some experience more modest results than the dramatic transformations seen in advertisements.

Ozempic has been studied at high doses for obesity treatment and has shown substantial weight loss effects. In clinical trials, it has demonstrated an average weight loss of around 15% or more of initial body weight in some individuals. This is compared to typically a 5% reported initial body weight with almost all other medications.

To separate the hype from reality, one needs only to turn to the real-life stories of those who have incorporated Ozempic into their diabetes management plans. These firsthand accounts provide a glimpse into the genuine impact of the medication.

Among those who found success with Ozempic, there are stories of individuals shedding significant pounds, feeling more energetic, and regaining a sense of control over their health. Many praise the medication for its role in helping them break free from the cycle of weight gain often associated with insulin therapy.

However, it would be remiss not to acknowledge those who do not experience such dramatic transformations. Ozempic is not always a magic pill, and its effects can vary. Some individuals find it challenging to tolerate the side effects, while others struggle to achieve substantial weight loss despite their best efforts. For them, the reality has not quite aligned with the soaring expectations.

Another crucial aspect to consider when evaluating Ozempic's impact is the role of lifestyle. While the medication can indeed assist in weight loss and blood sugar management, it is not a replacement for healthy living. Exercise, diet, and overall lifestyle choices remain pivotal in achieving and sustaining positive outcomes.

Ozempic is most effective when used as part of a comprehensive approach to diabetes management, one that emphasizes not only medication but also healthy habits. The reality is that sustainable weight loss and blood sugar control often requires a multifaceted strategy.

In the realm of medicine, hype often precedes reality. Ozempic, with its promise of weight loss alongside blood sugar control, is no exception. However, as the evidence has mounted and the experiences of patients and healthcare providers accumulates, it has became increasingly clear that

Ozempic is not just hype; it is a significant advancement in the treatment of diabetes and weight loss therapy.

But like all medical interventions, Ozempic is not a one-size-fits-all solution. Its effects vary, and its success depends on factors ranging from individual physiology to lifestyle choices. Thus, the reality of Ozempic lays in its potential to be a powerful tool in the arsenal against diabetes and weight loss, but it is not a panacea.

In the chapters that follow, we will continue to explore the nuances of Ozempic's impact, the science behind its mechanisms, and the broader implications of its place in the world of diabetes treatment. For now, one thing remains clear: Ozempic is no mere hype; it is a tangible reality, offering newfound hope and possibilities to those living with diabetes.

2

The Hype

The fascination surrounding Ozempic has reached remarkable heights, igniting a significant stir in its wake. It resonates less like a Hollywood blockbuster and more like a pivotal medical breakthrough. To put it simply, Ozempic is not your conventional Hollywood diet trend, even though some celebrities have adopted it as their clandestine weapon for shedding excess weight at an astonishing pace. Numerous celebrities now casually drop phrases like "Ozempic, darling" into conversations, as if it were the latest fashion accessory.

However, it's imperative to recognize that Ozempic and its counterpart, Wegovy, are not intended for the casual weight-watchers among us. Their purpose is geared towards individuals treading in the territory of extreme obesity, those whose health risks are substantially elevated due to their excessive weight.

One might wonder, "What's the harm in allowing those with a bit of extra weight to try it?" The issue arises from the Ozempic and Wegovy hype causing a worldwide shortage of these medications. Imagine a scenario where individuals genuinely requiring these drugs for critical health reasons are forced to wait in line behind trend-chasers, causing delays in accessing essential treatment.

Furthermore, this Hollywood-like saga takes a turn when medications are used for unintended purposes, leading to potential medical risks lurking in the background. It's akin to attempting to transform a romantic comedy into a horror film—things can become quite chaotic.

A Beverly Hills doctor closely associated with the health and beauty world notes, "Everyone's on it!" Ozempic has risen to superstardom in recent years due to its remarkable ability to accelerate weight loss. However, it achieves this by curbing one's appetite to the point where even the thought of indulging in tempting foods becomes a nauseating experience. It could be thought of as a behavioral psychologist's dream come true—mind over cravings, a real-life "A Clockwork Orange" for junk food enthusiasts.

On TikTok, videos showcasing Ozempic-assisted weight loss have gone viral, garnering views that make one wonder if the entire world is giving it a try. And the internet is abuzz with rumors suggesting Ozempic's involvement in the dramatic body transformations of celebrities. Some musicians and actors have discreetly hinted that they know A-listers who have embraced Ozempic, but these secrets remain as tightly guarded as the vault at Fort Knox.

Even the world's wealthiest individual, Elon Musk, doesn't shy away from praising this wonder drug, Ozempic. "Fasting + Ozempic/Wegovy + no tasty food near me," said the Chairman of X and Tesla.

Ozempic advertisements on television are inescapable, featuring individuals who have successfully managed their blood sugar levels and are savoring life to the fullest. They turn to the camera, their eyes brimming with excitement, while the soundtrack serenades us with the nostalgic melody of "Magic" by the Scottish rock group Pilot. "Oh! Oh! Oh! Ozeeeeempic!"

However, here's the twist: the weight loss aspect is mentioned almost as an afterthought. Amidst the rapid-fire recitation of precautions and potential side effects typical in pharmaceutical ads, the voice over casually drops, "You may lose weight!" To which a cheerful character responds, "Oh!"

The reason behind this casual approach is clear: Ozempic isn't strutting the catwalk as a weight loss sensation. No, it's positioning itself as a superhero among diabetes medications. It has garnered widespread acclaim in the medical community for its effectiveness in controlling blood sugar levels, often resulting in life-changing improvements for patients. But here's the intriguing part: it also reduces the desire to snack. Consequently, doctors are increasingly prescribing Ozempic off-label, solely for its ability to aid in weight loss.

However, let's not mistake Ozempic for a magic wand. Its wizardry lies in its ability to mimic a hormone called GLP-1, which plays a crucial role as the regulator of blood sugar levels. More about this later. When blood sugar levels rise, GLP-1 signals the body to produce more insulin rapidly, thus lowering those sugar levels. Moreover, GLP-1 has the remarkable ability to slow down the passage of food from the stomach to the small intestine, leading to a quicker sensation of fullness and reduced appetite.

Data from The Mayo Clinic reveals that when combined with a healthy lifestyle, weekly Semaglutide injections (the active ingredient in Ozempic) result in an average weight loss of approximately 33.7 pounds over 68 weeks.

The drug's popularity, coupled with its impressive results, has triggered a global rush to obtain it. However, there's a catch. The off-label use of Ozempic for weight loss is causing shortages for those who depend on it to manage type 2 diabetes.

Despite claims otherwise, we definitely live in an era of Ozempic shortage. Many of my patients are having trouble getting it from pharmacies. Some have turned to mail-order and internet sources, including "compounding" pharmacies and off-shore suppliers.

In the spring, the manufacturer of Ozempic, the Danish pharmaceutical giant Novo Nordisk, reported difficulties in meeting the surging demand. In Australia, recommendations were issued to prioritize Ozempic's use for on-label treatment of type 2 diabetes. As Australian authorities pointed out, "The shortage significantly affects people using Ozempic for its approved use."

The U.S. Food and Drug Administration (FDA) has sounded a similar alarm, attributing "intermittent supply disruptions" of certain Ozempic doses to a "demand increase for the drug." Reports are that the drug is on back order in some states until 2024.

Responding to the uptick in off-label prescriptions, Novo Nordisk intro-duced a new, rebranded drug called Wegovy. It is chemically identical to

Semaglutide but offered at higher doses, specifically targeting obesity and weight management. Now, Wegovy itself is facing a shortage. The FDA reports a temporary halt in the distribution of Wegovy in various dosages. The manufacturer has ceased shipments of the two smaller starter dose strengths until their manufacturing and supply chains can catch up with demand.

In 2013, the American Medical Association officially voted to declare obesity a disease, which demands both treatment and prevention efforts. The decision came after decades of debate, regarding whether obesity *was* a proper disease, or merely a behavioral issue, or a "lifestyle choice".

Despite the official declaration, and resulting changes in treatment protocols, the idea that being overweight is somehow a moral failing lingers in the culture. Some insurers have also denied coverage for GLP-1s, maintaining that weight loss treatments are a form "vanity." "Is obesity a medical condition that warrants treatment, or some sort of willpower issue?" Boyd asks, rhetorically. "We fundamentally believe that it is a medical issue that warrants treatment."

Desperate times may well call for desperate measures. But not everyone sees Ozempic (or Wegovy, or similar drugs) as some magical, miracle intervention into the obesity epidemic. But this miracle comes with its own costs, both medical and cultural.

Among the less common side effects are hair loss, heartburn and swelling at the site of injection. Others are even more severe. Animal studies have linked Semaglutide to an increased risk for thyroid cancers, as well as pancreatitis and gallstones. (Some law firms already seem to be gearing up to file suits on the basis of these adverse effects.) The drug's defenders would argue that such risks are acceptable, given the wide range of dangers associated with obesity: heart disease, stroke, sleep apnea, cancer, osteoarthritis and, of course, type 2 diabetes.

The broader cultural implications of injecting Semaglutide for weight loss are themselves wide-ranging. The link between obesity (or fitness) and "lifestyle" is tough to shake, despite the latest recommendations of doctors and medical authorities. Losing weight is typically regarded as an accomplishment: the result of hard work, dedication and tremendous self-discipline. (Such attitudes, which equate body weight to some sense of morality, may only work to reinforce the psychological bases of some eating disorders.) Does one show off their swollen injection site, as they might a newly sculpted six-pack of abdominal muscles? Does it make sense to congratulate someone for dropping 30lbs from taking Semaglutide? And what if they're doing so at the expense of putting people who may be more in need of the drug – such as type 2 diabetics – at further risk? And how is this weight loss going to be sustained when they stop taking Ozempic?

We will address these questions and many more in the chapters to follow.

II

The Science of Slim

3

The Discovery of Ozempic

The history of diabetes treatment is a long and evolving journey that has seen significant advancements over the centuries. Diabetes has been recognized since ancient times. Ancient Egyptians described a condition resembling diabetes in their medical texts. In the first century AD, the Greek physician Aretaeus of Cappadocia coined the term "diabetes" (meaning "siphon" in Greek) to describe excessive urination, a common symptom of the condition.

In ancient times, dietary modifications were the primary treatment for diabetes. Even ancient physicians and healers recommended diets low in carbohydrates and high in fiber. At the turn of the 20th century, these dietary recommendations still remained in place. Fasting and starvation diets were also found to manage diabetes: but these approaches often proved ineffective and harmful.

The most significant breakthrough in diabetes treatment came in 1921 when Canadian scientists Sir Frederick Banting and Charles Best discovered insulin. Their discovery revolutionized diabetes care by providing an effective treatment for type 1 diabetes, which was previously a fatal disease.

Before insulin was discovered, a person with diabetes could expect to suffer from a significantly increased risk of heart disease, stroke, andsama hypertension. Diabetes also commonly causes kidney damage, eye problems including blindness, nerve damage and circulatory problems. These complications can result in limb amputation. Uncontrolled blood sugar- the hallmark of diabetes- leads to mental confusion, and sometimes even coma.

Insulin is a hormone produced by the pancreas that regulates blood sugar levels. The ability to administer insulin via injections allows people with diabetes to survive and manage their condition.

In the 1950s and 1960s, researchers developed the first oral medications for diabetes management, including sulfonylureas and biguanides (metformin). These drugs work by different mechanisms than insulin, such as stimulating the body's own insulin secretion and reducing glucose production by the liver.

The development of portable blood glucose meters in the 20th century allowed people with diabetes to monitor their blood sugar levels more effectively. This technology enabled better self-management of diabetes through regular blood sugar testing. In recent years, continuous glucose monitoring devices allow for people to check their blood sugar from minute to minute - providing instant feedback and better control.

Originally, insulin was given to people in glass syringes. This has evolved to more convenient insulin pens and insulin pumps, innovations that improve the accuracy and ease of insulin administration.

During the last 40 years, new classes of medications for diabetes management, including thiazolidinediones, alpha-glucosidase inhibitors, GLP-1 receptor agonists, and DPP-4 inhibitors, were developed. These drugs offer alternative approaches to managing blood sugar levels and have expanded treatment options for individuals with diabetes.

The 21st century has also seen the emergence of advanced technologies, such as CGM systems and closed-loop insulin delivery systems, which offer real-time monitoring and automated insulin delivery. Ongoing research is exploring potential cures for diabetes, including stem cell therapies and the development of fully functional artificial pancreas systems. Advances in genetics and personalized medicine are leading to more tailored approaches to diabetes treatment, with a focus on individualized therapy plans.

The history of diabetes treatment reflects the continuous efforts of researchers, healthcare providers, and individuals with diabetes to improve care, enhance quality of life, and ultimately find a cure for this complex and challenging condition. Today, diabetes management involves a combination of medications, lifestyle modifications, and advanced technologies to achieve optimal blood sugar control and prevent complications.

The discovery of Ozempic is part of the broader history of glucagon-like peptide-1 receptor agonists (Incretins) and their development for the treatment of diabetes.

The story begins with the discovery of glucagon-like peptide-1 (GLP-1), a hormone produced in the gut in response to food intake. GLP-1 plays a crucial role in regulating blood sugar levels by stimulating *insulin release and inhibiting glucagon* secretion. These hormones are called incretins.

Researchers often look to nature for inspiration in drug discovery. In the case of GLP-1, they found inspiration from certain animals, including the angel fish and the Gila monster. Angelfish, also known as zebrafish, have a version of GLP-1 that shares some similarities with the human hormone. Scientists studied these fish to better understand the role of GLP-1 in regulating glucose metabolism.

The Gila monster is a venomous lizard found in the southwestern United States and Mexico. Researchers discovered that Gila monster saliva contains a substance called exendin-4, which is similar in structure and function to human GLP-1. Exendin-4 became the basis for the development of the first incretin analog studied in humans.

In the 1990s, researchers started exploring the potential therapeutic use of GLP-1 to treat diabetes. However, native GLP-1 has a very short half-life in the body, making it unsuitable for use as a medication.

To overcome the short half-life issue, scientists began developing synthetic incretin receptor agonists that mimic the effects of a person's normal GLP-1, which is released naturally in the human gut in response to food intake. Scientists sought to find a drug with a longer duration of action. These drugs would then mimic the action of GLP-1. These drugs were designed to be injected and stimulate insulin production in response to elevated blood sugar levels.

Exenatide (Byetta), based upon the molecule found in Gila monster saliva, was one of the first incretins to receive FDA approval in 2005. It marked the beginning of a new era in diabetes treatment, as it offered better blood sugar control with fewer hypoglycemic episodes and weight loss benefits. Other incretin analogs are also used that can be delivered daily or weekly, depending on their half-life.

Rational design led to the development of long-acting incretin analogs, such as semaglutide. This has had profound implications for the management of T2D in terms of improvements in glycemic control, body weight, blood pressure, lipids, beta-cell function, and CV outcomes.

Semaglutide, the active ingredient in Ozempic, was developed by Novo Nordisk, a Danish pharmaceutical company with a long history of diabetes research. Semaglutide is a long-acting GLP-1 RA that only needs to be injected once a week, improving patient compliance compared to daily injections

Semaglutide underwent extensive clinical trials to evaluate its safety and efficacy in managing blood sugar levels and promoting weight loss in people with type 2 diabetes. In December 2017, the US FDA approved Ozempic for the treatment of type 2 diabetes in adults. It became one of the latest additions to the incretin analogue class of medications.

Since its approval, semaglutide has been studied and developed for various applications, including the treatment of obesity. A higher-dose version of semaglutide, marketed as Wegovy, was approved by the FDA for chronic weight management in adults with obesity in 2021.

Ozempic and other incretin analogs have provided significant advance-ments in the management of type 2 diabetes, offering better glycemic control, weight loss benefits, and lower risks of hypoglycemia compared to some other diabetes medications. These discoveries represent a significant milestone in the ongoing quest to improve the lives of people living with diabetes

These discoveries illustrate the innovative ways in which researchers draw inspiration from nature to develop new medications for chronic conditions like diabetes. By studying the natural counterparts of human hormones, scientists have been able to create synthetic analogs that help individuals with diabetes better manage their condition and improve their overall health.

Through extensive research over the past 15 years, incretins have been found to be hormones that play a significant role in regulating blood sugar levels and the overall control of glucose metabolism. They are primarily produced and released by

cells in the gastrointestinal tract in response to the ingestion of food. Incretins help to fine-tune the body's insulin response and maintain blood sugar homeostasis.

GLP-1 is secreted by special cells in the small intestine in response to the presence of nutrients, especially carbohydrates. Stimulates the release of insulin from the pancreas in response to elevated blood sugar levels. This helps lower blood sugar after meals. GLP-1 also inhibits the release of glucagon, a hormone that raises blood sugar levels. It also slows down gastric emptying, which can help control post-meal blood sugar spikes. And it promotes a feeling of fullness or satiety, which may help regulate food intake and body weight.

In individuals with type 2 diabetes, the incretin system may not function optimally. As a result, the body may not release enough GLP-1 to control blood sugar levels effectively. Further understanding and manipulating the incretin system will lead to the development of other innovative therapies for diabetes management and weight control.

4

Understanding Insulin Resistance

Insulin resistance is a metabolic condition in which the body's cells become less responsive to the effects of insulin, a hormone produced by the pancreas. Insulin plays a crucial role in regulating blood sugar (glucose) levels by helping with the uptake of glucose from the bloodstream into cells, where it can be used for energy or stored for future use. When cells become resistant to insulin, it leads to several metabolic and health-related issues. Left untreated, insulin resistance can lead to full-blown diabetes.

There are several causes and risk factors for insulin resistance including obesity. Excess body fat, particularly abdominal fat, is a significant risk factor for insulin resistance. Combined with this is physical inactivity: A sedentary lifestyle contributes to insulin resistance and weight gain. But there are other factors that lead to insulin resistance that are not controllable such as genetics: Some individuals may have a genetic predisposition to insulin resistance; Age: Insulin resistance tends to increase with age, particularly after age 40; and conditions such as polycystic ovary syndrome (PCOS) and hormonal imbalances which can contribute to insulin resistance.

In insulin resistance, the body's cells, particularly muscle, liver, and fat cells, do not respond effectively to insulin's signaling. As a result, the pancreas produces more insulin to compensate. The consequences of insulin resistance are elevated blood sugar because cells cannot efficiently take up glucose from the bloodstream. This can lead to cardiovascular damage, high

22

blood pressure and cholesterol abnormalities.

Insulin resistance leads the pancreas to make more insulin to compensate for the poor glucose uptake. It is as if the body is signaling this important pancreas to churn out more hormone to fight an ever more difficult battle. After a while, the pancreas gives up - it surrenders and stops making insulin. The beta cells (the insulin-producing cells in the pancreas) start to shrink and die. When insulin production stops, the body no longer can compensate for increased blood sugar and irreversible diabetes sets in and insulin is usually required.

Most patients are diagnosed with diabetes long before needing insulin. The blood sugar is usually elevated and controlled with various oral medications for years before this "no turning back" event. But sadly, some of the conventional diabetes medications may hasten this event by putting even more pressure on the pancreas.

In addition to this insulin resistance can contribute to weight gain, making it challenging to lose excess weight. In some women, insulin resistance is often present in women with polycystic ovary syndrome and can contribute to fertility issues and hormonal imbalances.

It's important to note that insulin resistance is a manageable condition. Early detection and intervention through lifestyle changes and, if necessary, medications can help individuals with insulin resistance maintain better control of their blood sugar levels and reduce the risk of developing type 2 diabetes and associated health complications.

As clinicians have recognized insulin resistance as a precursor to diabetes, several approaches have been found to help: Lifestyle modifications are the primary approach to managing insulin resistance. This includes regular physical activity, a healthy diet, weight management, and stress reduction. In some cases, healthcare providers may prescribe medications to help improve insulin sensitivity or lower blood sugar levels. These may include metformin or insulin sensitizers. Achieving and maintaining a healthy weight can significantly improve insulin sensitivity. This comes from a balanced diet with an emphasis on whole foods, fiber, and controlled carbohydrate intake can help manage insulin resistance. And doctors have recognized that chronic stress can worsen insulin resistance. Stress-reduction techniques, such as mindfulness or relaxation exercises, can be beneficial.

Insulin resistance can have significant effects on the cardiovascular system, kidneys, and circulation, increasing the risk of several health issues.

Insulin resistance is strongly associated with an increased risk of cardiovascular diseases, including coronary artery disease, heart attacks (myocardial infractions), and strokes. This increased risk is due to various factors, including elevated blood sugar levels, high blood pressure, and abnormal lipid profiles.

Insulin resistance can contribute to high blood pressure, which is a major risk factor for heart disease and stroke. It often accompanies insulin resistance and worsens cardiovascular risk.

Insulin resistance is associated with an unhealthy lipid profile characterized by elevated levels of triglycerides and lower levels of "good" HDL cholesterol. This is different from the traditional cholesterol pattern where "bad" LDL is high. Both types of lipid abnormalities increase the risk of atherosclerosis (narrowing of the arteries).

Insulin resistance and high blood sugar levels can damage the small blood vessels in the kidneys, leading to a condition called diabetic nephropathy. Over time, this can result in reduced kidney function and even kidney failure. Diabetic nephropathy can lead to proteinuria, which is the presence of excess protein in the urine. It's an early sign of kidney damage in people with diabetes and insulin resistance.

Insulin resistance is associated with the development of atherosclerosis, a condition in which fatty deposits (plaques) accumulate inside the arteries. This narrows the arteries and reduces blood flow. Atherosclerosis can affect various parts of the circulatory system, including the coronary arteries (leading to heart disease) and the arteries in the legs (leading to peripheral artery disease).

As insulin resistance progresses, it can impair the ability of blood vessels to relax and dilate in response to changes in blood flow. This can lead to reduced blood flow to various organs and tissues.

Individuals with insulin resistance should work closely with their healthcare providers to develop a comprehensive plan for managing their condition and reducing the associated risks to their heart, kidneys, and circulation.

So it is now well known that insulin plays a pivotal role in regulating blood sugar levels by promoting glucose uptake into cells, where it can be used for energy or stored for future use. This hormone helps to prevent hyperglycemia (high blood sugar) and maintains glucose homeostasis throughout the day. Dysregulation of insulin production or function can lead to conditions such as type 1 diabetes (insulin deficiency) or type 2 diabetes (insulin resistance), which require medical management to maintain blood sugar control.

5

Hunger and Satiety

The regulation of hunger and satiety (the feeling of fullness) is a complex physiological process that involves various hormones, neural signals, and psychological factors. The goal is to maintain energy balance by ensuring that the body receives the necessary nutrients and calories to function properly.

Leptin and ghrelin are two hormones that play key roles in regulating hunger, appetite, and body weight. They have opposing effects on appetite and energy balance, and their interaction helps maintain homeostasis in the body. Here's an overview of leptin and ghrelin:

Leptin is often referred to as the "satiety hormone" or the "fat hormone" because it is produced by fat cells and released into the bloodstream in proportion to the amount of body fat. Its primary role is to signal to the brain that the body has sufficient energy stores and is not in need of additional food. Leptin **is p**roduced by fat cells. When fat stores increase, leptin levels rise and signal the brain to reduce hunger and increase energy expenditure. This helps maintain a stable body weight by preventing overeating.

In some individuals, a condition known as leptin resistance can occur. This means that despite high levels of leptin, the brain does not respond appropriately to its signals, leading to persistent feelings of hunger and potential weight gain.

Ghrelin is often called the "hunger hormone" because it is primarily produced by the stomach when it is empty and released into the bloodstream.

Ghrelin levels increase before meals and decrease after eating. Ghrelin acts on the hypothalamus to stimulate appetite and increase food intake. It triggers sensations of hunger, encourages meal initiation, and promotes energy storage in the body. Ghrelin secretion follows a circadian pattern, with higher levels typically observed in the evening and during fasting periods.

So clearly, leptin and ghrelin have opposing effects on appetite and energy balance. Leptin decreases appetite and promotes a feeling of fullness, while ghrelin stimulates appetite and increases hunger. This interplay helps regulate energy intake and expenditure in response to the body's energy needs. When energy stores are low (low leptin, high ghrelin), hunger is stimulated to encourage food consumption. Conversely, when energy stores are sufficient (high leptin, low ghrelin), appetite is suppressed.

Besides body fat levels, other factors can influence leptin and ghrelin levels. For example, sleep deprivation, stress, and certain dietary patterns can impact these hormones. Leptin and ghrelin have implications for understanding obesity, eating disorders, and metabolic disorders. Research into these hormones has led to the development of potential treatments for conditions related to appetite dysregulation. Some medications and interventions are being studied for their potential to modulate leptin and ghrelin levels to aid in weight management and appetite control.

While leptin and ghrelin are key players in the regulation of appetite and body weight, it's important to note that appetite control is a complex process involving multiple hormones, neural signals, and psychological factors. The balance between these various factors ultimately influences an individual's eating behavior and overall metabolic health.

The gastrointestinal tract communicates with the brain through neural pathways and hormonal signals. When food is ingested, stretch receptors in the stomach signal fullness to the brain. The gut signals the brain to regulate appetite and control hunger and satiety. Stretch receptors in the stomach detect food intake and send signals to the brain to stop eating when full. Fluctuations in blood sugar levels can influence hunger and satiety. After a meal, blood sugar levels rise, leading to feelings of fullness. Conversely, low blood sugar levels can trigger hunger.

The enteric nervous system, often called the "second brain," is a network of neurons embedded in the lining of the GI tract. It can operate independently of the central nervous system but also communicates with it. The vagus nerve, a major part of the parasympathetic nervous system, plays a central role in gut-brain communication. It sends sensory information from the GI tract to the brain and transmits signals from the brain back to the gut, regulating functions like digestion and satiety.

Hormones produced by the GI tract, such as cholecystokinin (CCK), ghrelin, and peptide YY (PYY), travel through the bloodstream to the brain. They convey information about food intake, nutrient absorption, and hunger/satiety.

The gut is home to a significant portion of the body's immune cells. Immune factors and inflammatory signals produced in the gut can affect brain function and may play a role in conditions like irritable bowel syndrome (IBS) and certain mood disorders. Gut microbiota, the trillions of microorganisms living in the intestines, interact with the immune system and may influence gut-brain communication. Emerging research suggests that the gut microbiota can have an impact on mental health and cognitive function.

Emotional states, stress, and psychological factors can influence gut function and vice versa. Stress can lead to changes in gut motility, permeability, and sensitivity, potentially exacerbating GI symptoms.

The circadian rhythms of blood sugar are tightly regulated by the body's internal clock and can impact overall metabolic health. Cortisol, a stress hormone, follows a circadian pattern with the highest levels typically in the morning and the lowest at night. Cortisol can influence blood sugar levels by promoting the release of glucose from the liver (gluconeogenesis). Insulin, which regulates glucose uptake by cells, also follows a circadian rhythm. Insulin sensitivity tends to be higher during the day and lower during the night.

Eating patterns and meal timing can impact blood sugar levels. Typically, blood sugar tends to be lowest in the morning after an overnight fast (fasting blood glucose) and rises after meals. The body's response to glucose differs throughout the day, with post-meal glucose spikes typically being more significant in the evening compared to the morning.

Circadian disruptions, such as shift work, irregular sleep patterns, or jet lag, can lead to disturbances in blood sugar regulation. This can increase the risk of insulin resistance, metabolic syndrome, and type 2 diabetes. Individuals with type 2 diabetes may experience higher blood sugar levels in the morning due to reduced insulin sensitivity (dawn phenomenon) or overnight hypoglycemia followed by rebound hyperglycemia (Somogyi effect).

The suprachiasmatic nucleus, located in the brain's hypothalamus, acts as the body's master clock. It receives input from light-sensitive cells in the retina and coordinates circadian rhythms. The SCN influences the release of hormones like melatonin and cortisol, which, in turn, impacts blood sugar regulation. While circadian rhythms follow a general pattern, there are individual variations. Some people may be "night owls" with delayed circadian rhythms, while others are "morning larks" with earlier rhythms.

Adequate and quality sleep is essential for maintaining healthy circadian rhythms and blood sugar regulation. Sleep deprivation and poor sleep quality can disrupt these rhythms and increase the risk of metabolic disorders. Chrononutrition is a field of study that explores how meal timing and the alignment of food intake with circadian rhythms can impact health. Some research suggests that aligning meals with the body's natural rhythms may have metabolic benefits.

Factors such as food preferences, portion sizes, and meal timing can influence hunger and satiety. Cognitive processes, like mindfulness and the anticipation of a meal, also impact eating behavior. Emotional states can affect appetite. Stress, for example, can lead to increased or decreased eating in different individuals.

The type of food consumed can affect satiety. Meals rich in fiber, protein, and healthy fats tend to promote feelings of fullness and sustained energy. Social situations, cultural norms, and the environment in which meals are consumed can influence eating behavior and satiety. Over time, repeated exposure to the same foods can lead to habituation, where the brain's response to a particular food diminishes, potentially reducing the sensation of fullness.

The body continuously monitors its energy stores and adjusts hunger and satiety signals accordingly. This is achieved through intricate feedback loops involving hormones and neural pathways. Certain medical conditions, such as hormonal imbalances, may disrupt the body's hunger and satiety regulation. For example, individuals with leptin resistance may not respond appropriately to the satiety signals sent by this hormone.

What about the incretin pathway we introduced in the prior chapter? New research has found an intricate relationship between incretins and leptin. Studies show that leptin may stimulate GLP-1 secretion from intestinal L cells, and leptin resistance may account for the decreased levels of GLP-1 found in obese humans.

The intricate balance between hunger and satiety constitutes a complex process that science will perpetually scrutinize and dissect. The progress made with GLP-1 agents represents another significant stride in comprehending the intricacies of eating physiology and metabolism, marking a crucial advancement in this field.

III

Ozempic

6

Getting Ozempic and Self-Injecting

As a physician, Ozempic and other incretin medications have become an important part of my toolbox of medications to fight diabetes and obesity. I have been in medical practice for more than 25 years. Back in the 1990s, all that physicians had to offer diabetics was insulin, metformin, and a class of medications called sulfonylureas. Each had its own limitations. Insulin requires injection, often many times per day. Although it is the most similar to the body's own hormones, it requires injection. Metformin can cause liver and kidney damage and is often associated with gastrointestinal discomfort. And sulfonylureas, such as glipizide and glimeperide, push your pancreas further into disrepair even though they help restore sugar balance. They are associated with a risk of sudden and dangerously low blood sugars (hypoglycemia) and they cause weight gain!

Then in the 2000's, there was a vast change in the treatment of diabetes, culminating in the release of Ozempic. Now doctors have many different classes of medications to treat diabetes and Ozempic, with its concurrent weight loss properties, has become amongst the most important.

Sometimes a new diabetic can present to the doctor or emergency room with severe symptoms of dehydration, severely high blood sugars, and metabolic derangement. These patients are often admitted to the hospital, where they are given intravenous fluids and insulin and monitored closely for electrolyte shifts that can occur when the blood sugar is being corrected.

More frequently, the patient presents to the doctor with mild symptoms, and a decision must be made regarding therapy. Ozempic and incretins are not first-line treatments for diabetics. The most important thing is to assess symptoms, the hydration state of the patient, along with an assessment of blood work that includes electrolyte measurement, possibility of concurrent infection, kidney function, vision changes, and symptoms of peripheral neuropathy.

Most of the time, with mild diabetes, a patient is given "lifestyle modification" instructions - directions for carbohydrate reduction and increased physical activity. Patients often go into a "honeymoon" phase: They listen to these directives and they normalize or improve their blood sugar control for several months.

Unfortunately, this willingness to change lifestyle is often short-lived. Further, the disease process of diabetes and insulin resistance is difficult to reverse. Many patients come back after their second or third recheck with their blood sugars escalating again.

At this point, a medication is usually introduced. If the numbers are severe, this may mean more than one medication to start. Many diabetics also have cholesterol problems and hypertension and need medication or that as well. And we know that any single diabetic medication can bring down a patient's long-term diabetic control - that magic tracking number, known as the hemoglobin A1C, by 1-1.5 %. So if a patient's diabetes is very out of control, they may require more than one diabetic medication.

Many clinicians are using it "off-label" as the first treatment when a diabetic first crosses the line into diabetes and also needs weight loss. The advantage of Ozempic, and other incretin medications, is that it helps restore pancreatic function, along with causing weight loss. This reversal of the diabetic process can not be ignored. All other diabetic medications can help control blood sugar and therefore help with diabetic complications. Ozempic and similar medications can reverse the process.

We don't know how long such reversal occurs. Patients taking similar incretin medications which have been on the market for more than a decade can certainly reduce their need for other medications or eliminate them entirely. However, it is rare, but not impossible to see a patient come off of all medications as if their diabetes is cured.

Amongst the side effects of Ozempic treatment is an increased risk of pancreatitis as well as a rare possibility of thyroid C cell cancer. I always order blood work for pancreatic enzymes and serum calcitonin to get a baseline in patients before starting Ozempic. And I recheck these numbers when the patient stays on Ozempic as I monitor them.

The popularity and hype associated with Ozempic has led to massive amounts of prescriptions being filled for this medication. Patients are getting the medication online and through doctors who are not experienced or qualified to prescribe this medication or monitor it. This is a huge emerging problem. Please make sure you obtain your medication from a clinician who will closely monitor you and who has experience and knowledge in using Ozempic.

So if your doctor has not recommended the medication to you, how do you ask for it? I have observed patient requests for specific medications to have grown enormously with the growth of direct to consumer pharmaceutical marketing. The hype of Ozempic has pushed this even further.

Sometimes your doctor will tell you that Ozempic is not right for you. Certainly, you should discuss this reasoning with the doctor. Often the decision is because the medication is relatively new and not part of the clinical experience of an individual practitioner. Unfortunately, many doctors stick to the things they learned in school or in residency – making some doctors stick to a regimen than may be outdated.

Sometimes doctors might be reluctant to prescribe the medication because they feel that a patient will be reluctant to self inject. I feel confident in writing that Ozempic self injection is extremely easy and virtually painless. The needle is extremely tiny. Most people do not even feel it at all. Ozempic comes in an injector pen where the needle is hidden. And is pressed against the injection site, either on the leg or lower abdomen. Again, the needle is so small that most people do not feel the needle going in. Similarly, the medication is injected, and is going in, most people don't feel it. Sometimes there is a slight burn. This doesn't feel like a bee sting or anything like that.

The process is virtually painless. Sometimes a patient will say that it burns for a minute after the medication goes in.

Remember, this medication does not go into a blood vessel and is superficially injected under the skin. There is a minor difference between Ozempic and Wegovy in terms of the injector. Ozempic can be adjusted by dialing the dosage on the pen. The pen is then placed on the injection site, and a button is pushed to push the tiny needle down into the skin and deliver the medication. Wegovy on the other hand has injector pens with single-dose preloaded amounts. The pen is placed on the skin, and when the entire pen is pressed down, the needle activates and pushes the medication under the patient skin through an identical, tiny needle.

So, in my opinion, the injection should not be an impediment to taking Ozempic. As long as your doctor is monitoring you for side effects, medication, interactions and compliance, Ozempic becomes a very important part of the treatment protocol for diabetes, especially when weight loss is also necessary or required.

Of course, there are many patients who ask for Ozempic who do not have diabetes. Some of them have insulin resistance, but many do not. There are many patients who just want to lose a few pounds, perhaps for an upcoming event, or just be thinner. For obese patients, Wegovy, which contains the same ingredient as Ozempic, is authorized by the FDA. But this authorization is not just for a few pound weight loss.

It is important for me to stress that Ozempic and Wegovy are not meant for people who just want to lose a few pounds. There are many people who are getting the medication for this reason. Some of them have lost weight through other means, and have been caught up in the weight loss industry and concerned about their body image. Ozempic seems to be a new godsend for these people.

Let's not fool ourselves. Certainly, there are going to be many patients who will use Ozempic and similar for small amounts or temporary of weight loss. I always ask the patient. Is it worth the risk for serious side effects to achieve this goal?

And how about the semaglutide pill? It's called Rybelsis. It doesn't have as much power as the injections. The weight loss is significant less. Rybelsus is a daily pill and it has no individual FDA indication for weight loss.

The stories I hear in patients taking Ozempic are extremely varied. Patients report lots of different things and I see different things beyond the commonly described side effects.

First off are the behavioral changes. Patients report that they aren't "thinking" about food as much as they previously did. This is different than prior weight loss medications where hunger suppression was usually driven by feeling full or nauseous. People also describe that they feel less stressed about food and making food choices. This is a major issue for some people, partially brought on by the diet industry.

Ozempic use also seems to suppress the "hangry factor". That is, the behavioral mood change that occurs in people when they haven't eaten in a while or social or temporal cues indicate that it is time to eat. People often manifest mood changes including anxiety and aggression. Many people report that this dissipates with Ozempic use.

A doctor's discussion with a patient about weight loss is often complex. Sometimes patients do not want to address this subject, even when a doctor details the risk of obesity and being overweight. Some patients respond to warnings about "Pre-diabetes" and "pre-hypertension" Other patients respond to more real-life discussions about their functional limitations because of the extra weight. Some clinicians use motivational interviewing to discuss weight loss strategies.

Once the subject of weight loss has been started with your doctor, the discussion now typically includes Ozempic and incretins. Doctors and other clinicians need to be aware of the changes in the classification of obesity when evaluating patients and weight loss strategies. Because obesity was only classified as a chronic medical condition in 2012, it is incumbent on a patient to seek out a clinician who is comfortable and confident in weight loss management, especially when seeking Ozempic or other incretins as a therapeutic choice.

In addition, the rise in Ozempic has led to a rise in social media advertising for weight loss and quick televisit sessions for the medication. Please be wary of these ads and their practitioners. Heed my advice that Ozempic and similar agents are strong medications that can cause serious side effects, some of them even deadly. Make sure you have a long-standing relationship with your clinician.

Before embarking on any weight loss program, it's advisable to consult with an experienced healthcare provider. They can provide personalized recommendations, monitor progress, and help ensure that the chosen approach is safe and suitable for your specific needs and health goals.

7

How to Use Ozempic

Self-injection medications are medications that individuals can administer to themselves through injections, typically using a syringe, pen device, or autoinjector. These medications are designed for a variety of medical conditions and are prescribed by healthcare providers based on the specific needs of the patient.

But the use of self-injection medications is not new and there are many newer medications that utilize this delivery method. Many people with diabetes, both type 1 and type 2, use self-injection medications like insulin or GLP-1 receptor agonists (e.g., Ozempic) to manage blood sugar levels. Medications used to treat autoimmune conditions, such as rheumatoid arthritis, multiple sclerosis, and psoriasis, are often administered via self-injection. Some hormone replacement therapies, like testosterone or growth hormone, require self-injection. Certain fertility treatments involve self-administered injections of hormones to stimulate ovulation. Epinephrine autoinjectors (e.g., EpiPen) are used for emergency treatment of severe allergic reactions (anaphylaxis).

For self-injection, there are different mechanisms for medication delivery. Some medications are drawn up into a syringe and injected manually. **Pen Devices** are pre-filled with medication and often used for insulin and other injectables. They are user-friendly and allow for more precise dosing. Wegovy comes as an autoinjector pen. Autoinjectors are designed for ease of use and often used for medications like epinephrine. They automatically deliver the medication with a push of a button.

Patients are typically trained by healthcare providers on how to properly administer self-injection medications. This training includes techniques for safe and effective injections.

The choice of injection site can vary depending on the medication. Common sites include the abdomen, thigh, buttocks, and back of the upper arm. Proper rotation of injection sites is often recommended.

Proper storage of either Ozempic or Wegovy medication is essential to maintain its effectiveness. These medications require refrigeration, although they can be left out at room temperature for a limited amount of time.

Adherence to the prescribed injection schedule is crucial for the medication's effectiveness. Skipping doses or not following the prescribed instructions can impact treatment outcomes. Patients who self-administer Ozempic or Wegovy must have regular check-ups with their healthcare provider to monitor their condition including periodic laboratory tests and adjustment of their medication as needed.

Self-injection medications have significantly improved the management of various medical conditions and have become a routine part of treatment for many individuals.

Just like with injections in other areas of the body, it's important to rotate injection sites to avoid repeatedly injecting into the same spot. This helps prevent the development of lumps or skin irritation. Ozempic is typically administered using a small, thin needle designed for subcutaneous injections, which minimizes discomfort. If you choose to inject Ozempic into your buttocks, make sure to clean the skin thoroughly with an alcohol swab, pinch the skin to create a fold, and inject the medication into the fold of the skin. The absorption rate of the medication can vary depending on the injection site. It's important to follow your healthcare provider's guidance on injection sites to maintain consistent blood sugar control.

Prolonged fasting and Ozempic

Prolonged fasting refers to extended periods of time without caloric intake, typically lasting longer than 24 hours. During prolonged fasting, the body relies on stored energy sources, such as glycogen (stored glucose) and eventually fat, to meet its energy needs. This can have implications for individuals who are using medications like Ozempic (semaglutide) to manage type 2 diabetes.

Prolonged fasting can increase the risk of hypoglycemia (low blood sugar) in individuals with diabetes, especially those taking medications that lower blood sugar levels, like Ozempic. Ozempic is a glucagon-like peptide-1 (GLP-1) receptor agonist that helps regulate blood sugar levels by increasing insulin secretion and decreasing glucagon release. During prolonged fasting, when there is little or no food intake, these effects can become more pronounced, potentially leading to hypoglycemia.

The risk of hypoglycemia during prolonged fasting varies from person to person and depends on factors such as medication dosage, overall health, and the duration of fasting. Some individuals may experience low blood sugar levels more quickly than others when fasting.

If you are considering prolonged fasting and are taking Ozempic or any other medication for diabetes, it is crucial to discuss your fasting plans with your healthcare provider.

Continuous monitoring of blood sugar levels during fasting is essential. Be prepared to check your blood sugar regularly and have a plan in place for addressing hypoglycemia if it occurs. Ensure that you have access to a source of fast-acting carbohydrates, such as glucose tablets or gel, to treat low blood sugar if needed.

The duration of fasting can significantly impact its effects on blood sugar. Shorter fasts (e.g., intermittent fasting) may be more manageable for individuals with diabetes than prolonged fasts that last several days. If you plan to undertake prolonged fasting, especially for more extended periods, it is advisable to do so under medical supervision. Your healthcare provider can provide guidance on how to minimize risks and monitor your health. If you have concerns about managing your blood sugar during fasting, you may explore alternative fasting strategies, such as time-restricted eating or shorter intermittent fasts that are less likely to pose significant risks.

Ozempic and Wegovy both share the same active ingredient, semaglutide. However, there are some differences between the two drugs:

Ozempic: Ozempic is primarily indicated for the treatment of type 2 diabetes. It is a glucagon-like peptide-1 receptor agonist (GLP-1 RA) that helps lower blood sugar levels by increasing insulin release and decreasing glucagon secretion. Wegovy is specifically approved for weight management in adults with obesity or overweight individuals with at least one weight-related comorbidity (e.g., hypertension, type 2 diabetes) in addition to a reduced-calorie diet and increased physical activity. It is a higher-dose formulation of semaglutide designed for weight loss.

Ozempic is available in lower doses for diabetes management, typically administered once a week. Wegovy: Wegovy is available in a higher dose and is administered once a week for weight management. Wegovy, being a higher-dose formulation of semaglutide, has demonstrated more significant weight loss effects compared to Ozempic in clinical trials specifically focused on obesity treatment. Wegovy has shown an average weight loss of around 15% or more of initial body weight in some studies. Ozempic can also lead to weight loss, but its primary indication is diabetes management, and the weight loss effects are typically not as pronounced as with Wegovy.

Ozempic was initially approved by the FDA for the treatment of type 2 diabetes before it was investigated and used for weight loss. Wegovy was specifically developed and approved by the FDA for weight management and obesity treatment.

The choice between Ozempic and Wegovy would depend on an individual's specific medical condition, whether they have type 2 diabetes or obesity, and the goals of treatment. It's important for individuals to discuss their options with a healthcare provider who can provide guidance on the most suitable medication based on their needs and health status.

Hypoglycemia (low blood sugar) is generally not a common side effect of

Ozempic (semaglutide) and Wegovy (also semaglutide). These medications are more commonly associated with reducing blood sugar levels and lowering the risk of hyperglycemia (high blood sugar).

While GLP-1 receptor agonists themselves do not typically cause hypoglycemia, the risk of hypoglycemia can still be influenced by other factors, such as concurrent use of other diabetes medications, especially insulin or sulfonylureas. If used in combination with these medications, the risk of hypoglycemia may increase. People with diabetes can respond differently to medications, and individual responses may vary. Some individuals may experience low blood sugar if they use GLP-1 receptor agonists in conjunction with other medications that lower blood sugar.

The dosage and titration of GLP-1 receptor agonists are typically carefully managed by healthcare providers. Adjusting the dose based on individual needs and responses can help minimize the risk of hypoglycemia. Hypoglycemia risk can also be influenced by factors such as dietary habits, physical activity, and adherence to the prescribed treatment plan. Consistent monitoring and adherence to a healthcare provider's recommendations are essential.

It's important for individuals with diabetes to be aware of the signs and symptoms of hypoglycemia and to have glucose-raising treatments (e.g., glucose tablets or gel) readily available in case hypoglycemia does occur.

While GLP-1 receptor agonists are generally associated with a low risk of hypoglycemia, it's crucial for individuals with diabetes to have regular follow-up appointments with their healthcare provider to monitor blood sugar levels and adjust treatment plans as needed. Any concerns about hypoglycemia or medication side effects should be discussed with a healthcare provider to ensure safe and effective diabetes management.

Clinical Trials for Ozempic (Semaglutide) for Weight Loss

Weight loss clinical trials are research studies designed to evaluate the safety and effectiveness of various interventions for weight management. These trials may involve diet and lifestyle modifications, medications, medical devices, or surgical procedures.

The Semaglutide Treatment Effect in People with Obesity (STEP) program included several clinical trials that evaluated the use of Ozempic (semaglutide) for weight management in individuals with obesity or overweight with certain comorbidities. These trials provided valuable data on the effectiveness of Ozempic for weight loss.

In the STEP trials, participants who received Ozempic typically achieved significant weight loss. On average, individuals taking Ozempic once weekly lost between 5% and 15% of their initial body weight over a 24-68 week period, depending on the specific trial. These trials involved various patient populations, including those with obesity, overweight individuals with type 2 diabetes, and those without diabetes.

It's important to note that individual responses to Ozempic can vary. Some participants in the trials experienced more substantial weight loss, while others had more modest results. Factors such as starting weight, adherence to treatment, diet, and physical activity level can influence the degree of weight loss.

Ozempic has shown the potential for maintaining weight loss over an extended period, which is a crucial aspect of its effectiveness in managing obesity. In some cases, Ozempic may be used in combination with other weight management strategies, such as lifestyle modifications and counseling, to enhance its effects on weight loss.

Remember that Ozempic is typically prescribed to individuals with a BMI (Body Mass Index) of 30 or greater or to those with a BMI of 27 or greater who have at least one weight-related comorbidity (e.g., type 2 diabetes, high blood pressure). The goal of treatment is not only weight loss but also the improvement of overall health and the reduction of obesity-related health risks.

What Happens After I Stop?

Weight changes after stopping Ozempic (semaglutide) can vary from person to person and depend on various factors, including individual metabolism, dietary habits, physical activity, and overall health. The weight changes which may occur after stopping Ozempic are influenced by multiple factors, and individual responses can vary. Maintaining healthy lifestyle habits, including dietary choices and regular physical activity, is essential for preventing weight regain after discontinuing the medication. Healthcare provider guidance and ongoing support can be valuable during this transition to ensure long-term success in managing weight and overall health.

8

Ozempic and Cholesterol Levels

Individuals with insulin resistance or diabetes frequently display specific cholesterol profiles that may elevate the likelihood of cardiovascular complications. These profiles usually look very different than traditional "high Cholesterol" patients who typically have elevated LDL levels.

People with insulin resistance or type 2 diabetes may have elevated LDL cholesterol levels, commonly referred to as "bad" cholesterol. Insulin resistance can lead to an increase in the production of LDL cholesterol by the liver and a decreased ability of cells to remove LDL cholesterol from the bloodstream.

However, insulin resistance and diabetes can be associated with lower levels of HDL cholesterol, known as "good" cholesterol. Reduced HDL cholesterol is linked to impaired reverse cholesterol transport, which means less effective removal of cholesterol from blood vessel walls.

Insulin resistance and diabetes are often accompanied by high triglyceride levels. Elevated triglycerides are a common feature of metabolic syndrome, which often coexists with insulin resistance and increases the risk of heart disease. In prediabetes and metabolic syndrome, the body often has difficulty processing triglycerides efficiently, leading to elevated levels. High triglycerides are an independent risk factor for CVD and are closely linked to insulin resistance, which is common in prediabetes.

People with insulin resistance or diabetes may have a higher proportion of small, dense LDL particles, which are more atherogenic (more likely to contribute to plaque buildup in arteries) than larger, buoyant LDL particles. In addition to total LDL cholesterol, the number of LDL particles is an important marker. Having a high LDL particle number (small, dense LDL particles) is associated with an increased risk of CVD. Prediabetic individuals and those with metabolic syndrome may have an unfavorable LDL particle profile.

The combination of high LDL cholesterol, low HDL cholesterol, and elevated triglycerides creates an atherogenic lipid profile, increasing the risk of atherosclerosis and cardiovascular disease.

Managing cholesterol in people with insulin resistance or diabetes is critical for reducing the risk of heart disease and other cardiovascular complications.

It's crucial for individuals with insulin resistance or diabetes to work closely with their healthcare team, which may include endocrinologists, cardiologists, and registered dietitians, to develop a personalized plan for managing cholesterol and reducing cardiovascular risk. This plan should consider individual health factors and goals.

Low HDL (high-density lipoprotein), high triglycerides, and high LDL particle number are common lipid abnormalities often associated with prediabetes and metabolic syndrome. These abnormalities can contribute to an increased risk of cardiovascular disease (CVD). Here's an overview of each of these lipid abnormalities and their relationship with prediabetes and metabolic syndrome:

High LDL particle number, also known as high LDL-P or elevated LDL particle concentration, refers to an increased concentration of low-density lipoprotein (LDL) particles in the bloodstream. LDL particles are often categorized into two main types based on their size and density: small, dense LDL particles and large, buoyant LDL particles. When we refer to a high LDL particle number, it typically means an increase in the number of small, dense LDL particles, which is associated with an increased risk of cardiovascular disease (CVD).

We need to have a more detailed explanation of high LDL particle number and its significance on cardiovascular and cerebrovascular disease

First off, it is important to distinguish LDL particles from the the LDL measurement typically reported in a laboratory measurement of cholesterol. These are not the same measurements because LDL and LDL particles measure different things.

LDL particles are carriers of cholesterol in the bloodstream. They transport cholesterol from the liver to various cells and tissues in the body. LDL particles contain a core of cholesterol esters and a surface layer of lipids and proteins. The composition and size of these particles can vary. LDL is one of the atherogenic lipid species carried within the LDL particle.

Small, dense LDL particles are smaller and more compact than large, buoyant LDL particles. Small, dense LDL have less LDL carrying capacity and are more susceptible to oxidation and can penetrate the arterial wall more easily, contributing to the formation of atherosclerotic plaque.

Elevated LDL particle number, particularly an increase in small, dense LDL particles, is considered a significant risk factor for cardiovascular disease. These small particles are more atherogenic (more likely to contribute to atherosclerosis) than larger LDL particles. They are associated with an increased risk of plaque formation in the arteries, narrowing of blood vessels, and an elevated risk of heart attacks and strokes.

High LDL particle number can be influenced by various factors, including genetics, diet, lifestyle, and certain medical conditions. Common factors associated with high LDL particle number include a diet high in saturated and trans fats, insulin resistance, obesity, and metabolic syndrome.

High LDL particle number can be assessed through advanced lipid testing, such as nuclear magnetic resonance (NMR) spectroscopy or gradient gel elec-trophoresis. These tests provide information about the size and distribution of LDL particles.

Managing high LDL particle numbers involves comprehensive cardiovascu-lar risk reduction strategies, including reducing saturated and trans fats in the diet, regular physical activity, smoking cessation, and weight management. In some cases, healthcare providers may prescribe statins or other lipid-lowering medications to lower LDL particle number. For high small, dense LDL particles or a high LDL particle number, a doctor specializing in lipid and cholesterol management will prescribe insulin-sensitizing medications and sometimes omega-3 fatty acids. This will require regular follow-up with healthcare providers to assess lipid levels and cardiovascular risk.

Ozempic is one such agent that can cause insulin sensitization and shift the LDL particle abnormality. Multiple studies have shown that LDL particle number is a more important predictor of cardiovascular disease than LDL concentration (seen in basic lipid profiles), especially if there is a discordance in between these two measurements.

Thus a more thorough and comprehensive understanding of lipid abnormalities in diabetics, overweight individuals and insulin-resistant patients should prompt your doctor to think outside the one-size-fits-all method of statins for all high cholesterol problems. Patients with metabolic obesity, insulin resistance and diabetes often see their blood sugar numbers worsen with statin use. Although reduction of LDL concentration with statins is a mainstay of cardiovascular risk reduction, a more personalized and disease specific approach is usually necessary.

It's important to note that assessing and managing cardiovascular risk involves considering multiple factors beyond LDL particle number, including blood pressure, overall cholesterol levels, smoking status, and family history of heart disease. Healthcare providers use a combination of these factors to assess an individual's risk and develop personalized treatment plans to reduce the risk of cardiovascular events.

9

Cosmetic Changes and Self-Image

One of the primary effects of Ozempic is weight loss. Many people experience gradual weight loss while taking the medication. The amount of weight lost can vary but is often modest to moderate. Some individuals may experience more significant weight loss, particularly when Ozempic is combined with a healthy diet and regular exercise.

Ozempic can lead to a decrease in body fat percentage, which is beneficial for individuals with type 2 diabetes, as excess body fat can contribute to insulin resistance. As individuals lose weight on Ozempic, they may notice changes in their body composition. This may include a reduction in waist circumference and a more favorable distribution of body fat. Indeed, people with insulin resistance tend to have more abdominal fat or visceral fat and this weight usually can be shed when using Ozempic. Therefore a change in body shape usually comes with loss of abdominal girth. This change in body composition brought about by Ozempic may result in a slimmer appearance or smaller clothing sizes.

In some cases, weight loss on Ozempic may lead to improved muscle definition, especially if individuals engage in regular physical activity while taking the medication. People typically experience a slimmer overall appearance as they lose weight. Some individuals may notice changes in their facial appearance as weight is lost. This can include a more defined jawline and cheekbones. Weight loss on Ozempic can lead to changes in body proportions.

For example, individuals may find that their clothing fits differently, with a smaller size needed for tops or pants.

As individuals achieve their weight loss goals while taking Ozempic, they often experience increased confidence and a positive change in their self-image.

It's important to note that while many people experience these positive changes when taking Ozempic, individual responses can vary. Some individuals may not experience significant weight loss, and others may have different side effects. Additionally, lifestyle factors, such as diet and exercise, play a significant role in determining the extent of these changes.

One trial found that after 2 years on semaglutide, patients were still losing weight [5]. Although there is technically no limit to how long you can take Ozempic weekly, at we mostly recommend sticking with the medication for at least a year.

If you're not losing weight on Ozempic, there could be a few reasons why.

You're looking for drastic changes, quickly:

While Ozempic can help you experience significant weight loss, it does take time. Try to approach your journey with Ozempic as one to help you achieve gradual, sustainable weight loss.

You don't have the right calorie intake

It's still important to be in a caloric deficit to lose weight. That's why our programme uses behavioural science to set you up for sustainable lifestyle changes that will stick.

Your dosage might be off

It's required that you start on a dose of 0.25mg for the first 4 weeks, which allows your body to get used to the medicine and helps to reduce the risk of side effects.

After the initial 4 weeks, you can begin increasing the dosage — be sure to talk to your prescriber about this as you may not have increased your dose and that could be wreaking havoc with your weight loss efforts.

You've hit a plateau

It's normal to eventually hit a point where your weight loss slows down, especially if you're not working on keeping or building up your muscle mass.

Losing muscle along with fat slows your metabolism and can slow down your weight loss. Once your body adjusts, your weight loss journey should pick up again.

You haven't found the right healthy lifestyle changes

The true 'secret' to long-term weight management is being able to establish healthy habits like diet changes you can actually stick to long-term. This will ensure your weight loss is sustainable and continues into the future.

You need a stronger support network

Successful people surround themselves with successful people. How do people lose weight?

Research shows people have greater success with weight loss when they do it together.

You're not getting enough sleep

Getting at least 8 hours of sleep a night is critical to helping your body lose weight. Try to practice good sleep hygiene to ensure you're giving yourself the best opportunity for a good night's sleep.

Ozempic helps reduce cravings and suppress appetite, which helps you consume fewer calories. Each person has a different starting weight, metabolic weight and possibly even different underlying health conditions.

Once you start on an injectable medication, you may find it takes a few weeks to start seeing results, although some people may see changes in a week.

You will also start on a low dose to give your body time to slowly adjust to feel satisfied and not feel hungry. Once you use Ozempic, you should experience increased satiety, which helps your body to gradually adjust and begin to lose weight.

In general, most people lose a minimum of 5% of their starting weight when they use Ozempic.

Individuals with body dysmorphic disorder (BDD) may face unique challenges when taking medications like Ozempic (semaglutide) that can affect body weight and appearance. BDD is a mental health condition characterized by an obsessive focus on perceived flaws or defects in one's physical appearance, even if those flaws are minimal or nonexistent.

People with BDD may be particularly sensitive to changes in their physical appearance. Medications that lead to weight loss, such as Ozempic, can exacerbate body image concerns and trigger obsessive thoughts about their appearance.

Healthcare providers should be aware of a patient's history of BDD or body image issues. Regular monitoring and open communication are crucial. Patients should feel comfortable discussing any changes in their perception of body image.

BDD often requires psychological intervention, such as cognitive-behavioral therapy (CBT) or medication, to address obsessive thoughts and improve body image perception. Individuals with BDD may benefit from ongoing counseling or therapy in addition to diabetes management.

Healthcare providers should help individuals with BDD set realistic expectations for the effects of Ozempic. Weight loss should be viewed as a part of overall health management rather than an obsession with appearance.

Doctors should encourage individuals with BDD to seek support from mental health professionals and support groups focused on body image issues. These groups can provide a safe space for sharing experiences and coping strategies.

Treatment plans for individuals with both diabetes and BDD should be individualized. Balancing the need for diabetes management with concerns related to body image is essential.

It's crucial for individuals with BDD and their healthcare providers to work together as a team to address both their diabetes management and mental health needs. Open and honest communication about concerns related to body image and medication effects is essential to ensure the best possible care and support.

Addiction is a complex and multifaceted condition influenced by various factors, including genetics, psychology, environment, and social factors. Medications used in the treatment of addiction typically target specific neurotransmitter systems or receptors associated with the addictive substance.

Some individuals with type 2 diabetes may also struggle with alcohol dependence or misuse. In such cases, it's important for healthcare providers to consider the potential interactions between diabetes medications, alcohol consumption, and the management of both conditions.

Alcohol can lower blood sugar levels, which can be particularly concerning for individuals taking medications like Ozempic that also lower blood sugar. Combining alcohol with Ozempic may increase the risk of hypoglycemia (low blood sugar). It's essential to monitor blood sugar levels closely and avoid excessive alcohol consumption.

People can have varying responses to alcohol, and the effects can be unpredictable, especially when combined with medications. Some individuals may experience increased sensitivity to the effects of alcohol, while others may have reduced sensitivity.

Alcohol can interact with medications in various ways. It may affect the metabolism and effectiveness of certain drugs, although specific interactions with Ozempic are not well-documented.

: If you are taking Ozempic and have concerns about alcohol use or dependence, it's crucial to discuss these concerns with your doctor. They can provide guidance on safe alcohol consumption, potential interactions, and appropriate management of both conditions.

For individuals with alcohol dependence or misuse issues, a comprehensive treatment approach, which may include counseling, support groups, or addiction treatment programs, is typically recommended. Ozempic alone is not a treatment for alcohol dependence.

It's essential to be open and honest with your healthcare provider about your alcohol consumption and any concerns you have regarding its inter-action with your diabetes medication. They can help you make informed decisions and develop a personalized treatment plan that addresses both your diabetes management and any alcohol-related issues. Additionally, medical guidelines and research may have evolved since my last update, so consulting with a healthcare professional is essential for the most current information.

While Ozempic is safe to use with a doctor's recommendation, it can cause rapid weight loss that is often more pronounced on the face.

Facial fat serves a protective function and affects facial aesthetics and elasticity. Weight loss can cause dermatological changes and shrinking because the fat that stretches and cushions the skin is no longer in place.

The skin of the face also loses its ability to retract after an episode of rapid weight loss due to reduced levels of elastin and collagen, which are essential for structural integrity.

As a result, people taking Ozempic may report increased signs of aging, such as more lines and wrinkles, loss of fat, which can lead the skin to become loose and sag, a hollowed-out appearance and lipodystrophy, which affects how the body accumulates and stores fat

If a person takes Ozempic, they may be unable to prevent facial side effects. However, if these are a cause for concern, a doctor may recommend reducing the dosage, changing to a different medication, drinking 1–2 liters of water every day, improving protein intake with a protein-rich diet, using dermatological fillers and lifestyle modifications to maintain a healthy weight

If a person decides to stop taking Ozempic, it can take about 5 weeks from the last dose for the drug to clear from their system.

Lipodystrophy is a rare disorder that affects how the body accumulates and stores fat. There may be additional fat, for instance, around the abdomen and very little in others, such as the arms. Lipodystrophy is a disorder that affects how the body accumulates and stores fat. In a person with this condition, fat collects in certain areas, such as the torso, face, and neck, while the legs and arms have little to no fat.

What happens with fat loss with Ozempic use? Skin changes attributed to nutrition and vitamin depletion can manifest quite rapidly. This depletion often leads to the reabsorption and atrophy of fat, contributing to a prematurely aged and gaunt appearance. To better understand this process, envision a balloon filled with air: initially, releasing a small amount of air doesn't significantly affect its tightness. However, as more air escapes, the balloon becomes loose, and its elasticity can't compensate for the loss of volume. A similar mechanism occurs within the body and face. Our skin can adapt to weight fluctuations by stretching and recoiling, thanks to elastin fibers at the cellular level. However, as we age, our skin's capacity to contract diminishes, and we experience volume loss, ultimately leading to skin laxity.

Furthermore, lips can undergo changes, losing some of their fatty tissue bulk, particularly with age or weight loss. This reduction can result in a dehydrated or shrunken appearance. Some individuals embrace the loss of facial volume, while others perceive it as aging.

The phenomenon known as the "Ozempic face" has gained attention due to its rapid fat loss, causing facial skin to appear gaunt and aged. This has prompted many individuals to seek remedies from dermatologists and cosmetic surgeons, often involving costly procedures.

Commonly affected facial features include drooping cheeks, which may lead to slight indents and wrinkles at the temples, as well as sunken under-eye areas. The skin beneath the chin may also exhibit sagging in cases of substantial weight loss. To counteract the "Ozempic face," some practices turn to hyaluronic acid fillers like Restylane or Juvéderm to restore immediate volume loss. Additionally, secondary fillers such as Sculptra, an injectable poly-L-lactic acid, can stimulate collagen production and provide structural support over several weeks.

Interestingly, there is a growing trend of millennials using Ozempic, with some experiencing premature aging. These changes underscore the importance of understanding the effects of rapid fat loss on facial appearance and considering appropriate interventions to maintain a youthful look.

10

Exploring Potential Side Effects

Every medication has side effects. I often tell patients that if one were to read the potential side effects for aspirin, you would never take one! But if a side effect is predictable and can be monitored for, it usually means that a medication balances the good and the bad - resulting in health effect that is beneficial to the patient.

Sometimes side effects and toxicities emerge years or even decades after medication are used. This is always a concern and has been an issue in the past with some weight loss medications (Redux and FenPhen). So far, we know some predictable side effects with Ozempic. And some toxicities that make the medication not suitable for some patients.

All this underscores that Ozempic should be prescribed and monitored by a competent medical professional. On-line prescription mills and walk-in clinic prescribing is an absolute no-no for this medication. Ozempic can have profound effects on your organs. ANd this has to be closely monitored as you take the medication. And perhaps for a period of time once you stop it.

It's important to note that not everyone will experience these side effects, and some may experience them to a lesser degree.

Nausea is one of the most common side effects when starting Ozempic. It typically occurs during the initial weeks of treatment and tends to improve over time. It can reoccur when the dose is increased. In some people, they cannot tolerate the nausea or sometimes even vomiting and stop the medication.

Some people may experience a reduced appetite, which can contribute to weight loss. So this is really part of the therapeutic effect of the medication. But some people can experience hypoglycemia (Low Blood Sugar). While Ozempic itself does not usually cause hypoglycemia when used alone, it can increase the risk of low blood sugar when used in combination with other diabetes medications that lower blood sugar.

There may be mild irritation or redness at the Ozempic injection site . This is usually temporary and not a cause for concern.

Another side effect that is common and potentially troubling is constipation accompanied sometimes by abdominal pain. Part of the effect of Ozempic is to slow down the time that food moves through your intestines. Paradoxically, this leads to more efficient nutrient extraction as the food sits longer in you. Remember those Gila monsters and their saliva? Gila monsters typically eat a meal and sit for days or even weeks in the sun before eating again.

But Ozempic can also be associated with some more alarming and sometimes deadly side effects. In rare cases, pancreatitis (inflammation of the pancreas) has been reported as a side effect of Ozempic. Symptoms of pancreatitis include severe abdominal pain that may radiate to the back, nausea, and vomiting. If you experience these symptoms, you should seek immediate medical attention.

Diagnosing medication-induced pancreatitis typically involves a combination of medical history assessment, physical examination, blood tests to measure pancreatic enzyme levels, and imaging studies such as ultrasound, CT scans, or MRI. Treatment for medication-induced pancreatitis primarily involves discontinuing the medication suspected of causing the condition. Supportive care may be needed, including hospitalization for severe cases. Patients may require intravenous fluids, pain management, and nutritional support.

There have been reports of thyroid tumors, including thyroid cancer, associated with Ozempic use in animal studies. However, the risk of this side effect in humans is still being studied. These tumors are in the C cells of the thyroid, which make the hormone calcitonin (part of your calcium regulation.) I feel that pancreatic enzymes and calcitonin levels should be regularly monitored in patients taking Ozempic.

Calcitonin-producing tumors, also known as medullary thyroid carcinomas, are a type of neuroendocrine tumor that originates in the thyroid gland. These tumors are characterized by the overproduction of calcitonin, a hormone that helps regulate calcium levels in the body. Medullary thyroid cancers sometimes run as a cluster of cancers in some families and patients with their own history of thyroid cancer or any of the multiple endocrine neoplasia (MEN) tumors should not take Ozempic.

Symptoms to look for that might signal thyroid cancer in any patient include a palpable thyroid nodule or lump in the neck, swelling or enlargement of the thyroid gland, hoarseness or voice changes due to pressure on the vocal cords, difficulty swallowing, neck pain or discomfort and diarrhea (in advanced cases).

While rare, some people may experience allergic reactions to Ozempic. Signs of an allergic reaction may include rash, itching, swelling, severe dizziness, and difficulty breathing. Also seek immediate medical attention if you suspect an allergic reaction.

It's essential to use Ozempic as prescribed by your healthcare provider and to report any unusual or severe side effects to them promptly. Your healthcare team can help you manage side effects and determine if Ozempic is the right medication for you. Additionally, discuss your medical history and any other medications you are taking with your healthcare provider, as this can influence the risk of side effects.

Semaglutide, the active component of both Ozempic and Wegovy can interact with other drugs, potentially affecting their effectiveness or increasing the risk of side effects. It's crucial to inform your healthcare provider about all the medications, supplements, and over-the-counter drugs you are taking to avoid potential interactions.

There are some notable medication interactions with Semaglutide. These interactions can be categorized into those where Semaglutide is enhancing the effects of other diabetic medications. For example, Ozempic may enhance the glucose-lowering effects of oral diabetes medications such as sulfonylureas (e.g., glipizide, glyburide) or meglitinides (e.g., repaglinide). This can increase the risk of hypoglycemia (low blood sugar). Dosage adjustments may be necessary. Combining Ozempic with insulin may also increase the risk of hypoglycemia. Your healthcare provider may need to adjust your insulin dosage when using both medications.

The use of corticosteroids alongside Ozempic may affect blood sugar levels by counteracting the blood sugar-lowering effect of Ozempic.

Because Ozempic can slow down stomach emptying (gastric emptying) some other medications that depend on a specific rate of absorption in the stomach, such as certain antibiotics or oral contraceptives, may have their effectiveness reduced while taking Ozempic. Medications that influence gastrointestinal motility, such as anticholinergic drugs or opioids, may potentially interact with Ozempic by affecting the rate at which the medication is absorbed.

Other Ozempic drug interactions include an alteration of the metabolism of warfarin, a blood-thinning medication, potentially leading to changes in international normalized ratio (INR) values. Regular monitoring of INR is advisable when these medications are used together. Some medications that affect kidney function may interact with Ozempic. While Ozempic itself can have a blood pressure-lowering effect, it may interact with other medications used to treat high blood pressure. Also, some herbal supplements and alternative therapies may interact with Ozempic.

Remember that individual responses to medication interactions can vary, and your healthcare provider will consider your unique medical history and needs when making treatment decisions. Never stop or adjust your medication regimen without consulting your healthcare provider first, as this can lead to uncontrolled blood sugar levels or other health issues. Always communicate openly with your healthcare team about all medications you are taking.

Always consult with your healthcare provider before taking any medication while breastfeeding. They can assess your specific situation and provide guidance based on your medical history, the health of your baby, and the potential risks and benefits.

Your healthcare provider will weigh the potential risks associated with taking Ozempic against the benefits of managing your diabetes. They will consider whether the medication's benefits to you outweigh any potential risks to your breastfeeding infant.

Your healthcare provider may explore alternative treatment options for managing diabetes while breastfeeding. Some diabetes medications may be considered safer during breastfeeding than others. If you and your healthcare provider decide that continuing Ozempic while breastfeeding is the best course of action, close monitoring of your baby's health, blood sugar levels, and overall development may be necessary. Seek guidance from a lactation consultant or breastfeeding specialist to ensure proper breastfeeding techniques and optimal nutrition for your baby. The timing of Ozempic administration in relation to breastfeeding may be a consideration. Your healthcare provider may provide specific recommendations on when to take the medication in relation to breastfeeding.

11

Questions and Answers For Your Clinician/Doctor

Question 1: What is Ozempic, and how does it work?

Answer: Ozempic is a medication used to treat type 2 diabetes. It belongs to a class of drugs called GLP-1 receptor agonists. It works by mimicking the action of the hormone GLP-1, which helps regulate blood sugar levels. Ozempic stimulates insulin secretion, reduces glucagon production, slows stomach emptying, and promotes a feeling of fullness, ultimately leading to better blood sugar control.

Question 2: Is Ozempic suitable for my type 2 diabetes management, and why?

Answer: Whether Ozempic is suitable for your diabetes management depends on your specific medical history, current treatment regimen, and treatment goals. It's effective for many people with type 2 diabetes, particularly when diet and exercise alone aren't sufficient to control blood sugar. Your healthcare provider will assess your individual circumstances to determine if it's appropriate for you.

Question 3: How is Ozempic administered, and how often?

Answer: Ozempic is administered by subcutaneous injection, which means it is injected under the skin. It's typically injected once a week on the same day each week. The specific dosage and injection site will be discussed and prescribed by your healthcare provider.

Question 4: What potential side effects should I be aware of when taking Ozempic?

Answer: Common side effects of Ozempic may include nausea, vomiting, diarrhea, and abdominal pain. These side effects often improve with time. Serious but rare side effects can include pancreatitis, allergic reactions, and changes in kidney function. It's important to report any unusual symptoms or side effects to your healthcare provider.

Question 5: How can I manage potential side effects of Ozempic?

Answer: To manage common side effects like nausea, starting with a lower dose and gradually increasing it may help. Additionally, taking Ozempic with a meal can reduce gastrointestinal side effects. If you experience severe side effects or have concerns, it's essential to consult with your healthcare provider.

Question 6: Will taking Ozempic require adjustments to my other diabetes medications?

Answer: Depending on your current diabetes medication regimen, your healthcare provider may adjust your treatment plan when you start taking Ozempic. It's crucial to inform your provider about all medications you are taking to ensure compatibility and safety.

Question 7: How will Ozempic affect my blood sugar levels, and what should

I expect in terms of A1c reduction?

Answer: Ozempic is known to lower blood sugar levels. The extent of blood sugar reduction varies from person to person. Your healthcare provider will monitor your progress and make adjustments as needed to achieve your target A1c level.

Question 8: Can Ozempic help with weight loss?
   Answer: Yes, Ozempic has been associated with weight loss in many individuals. On average, people may lose between 5% and 15% of their initial body weight over several months. However, individual responses can vary.

Question 9: What are the long-term benefits and risks of taking Ozempic?

Answer: Ozempic has shown long-term benefits in terms of blood sugar control and potential weight loss. However, like any medication, it comes with potential risks, including side effects such as pancreatitis. Your healthcare provider will assess the benefits and risks specific to your situation.

Question 10: What lifestyle changes should I consider in conjunction with taking Ozempic?

Answer: A healthy diet and regular physical activity are essential components of diabetes management. Your healthcare provider will provide guidance on diet and exercise tailored to your needs. It's important to maintain a collaborative relationship with your healthcare team to optimize your treatment plan.

12

Questions To Ask Yourself

Here are some important issues you should think about:

Why Am I Being Prescribed Ozempic?

Understand the specific reasons your healthcare provider is recommending this medication and how it will help manage your diabetes and help with your weight loss. Do you have insulin resistance or diabetes? Are you metabolically obese? Sometimes your doctor may see other signs of obesity such as kidney insufficiency, hypertension, hypercholesterolemia, or high inflammatory markers. These can exist in someone with only a little weight to lose.

How Should I Take Ozempic?

Are you ready for self-injection? Can someone help yo with this You need to consider the correct dosage, injection technique, and when to take the medication. You should have a plan for dosing regimen, dosing escalation, timing, how to inject and where on your body to inject.

Are Am Aware And Capable Of Monitoring For Side Effects?

Inquire and understand the common as well as the rare side effects associated with Ozempic and what to do if you experience any of them. Your doctor should give you advice on follow-up testing and monitoring. And you should be diligent with these recommendations. One of the worst things you can do is take Ozempic with no medical followup.

Will Ozempic Affect My Blood Sugar Levels?

Learn how Ozempic works to lower your blood sugar and how it should be integrated into your overall diabetes management plan. Ask how it interacts with other medications you may be taking. Talk to your doctor about modifying other medications, if necessary.

What Are the Benefits of Ozempic for me?

Discuss the potential benefits of using Ozempic, including improvements in blood sugar control, weight loss, and other health outcomes. Below, we discuss the positive and negative financial aspects of taking Ozempic. Consider these before embarking on Ozempic treatment.

What Should I Do If I Miss a Dose?

Understand the protocol for missed doses. You should never "double up" your dose. Have a plan and in place if you miss a dose or are delayed. As we write this book, many pharmacies are having trouble keeping Ozempic in stock. Speak to your doctor about what to do in case you have started Ozempic and are unable to obtain refills.

Can I Combine Ozempic With My Current Diabetes Medications?

If you're already taking other diabetes medications, ask your doctor or pharmacist if Ozempic can be used in combination with them and if any adjustments may be necessary.

Is Ozempic Safe For Me As A Women of Childbearing Age?

If applicable, discuss the safety of Ozempic during pregnancy with your doctor and whether effective contraception is needed. Your doctor must be able to give you adequate advice regarding Ozempic during pregnancy and breast-feeding.

Are There Any Interactions with Other Medications or Supplements I'm Taking?

Inquire about potential drug interactions with other medications or supplements you are currently using. Not just diabetes medications. Make sure your doctor knows all the medications you are taking as well as the dosages.

What Lifestyle Changes Should I Make Alongside Ozempic?

Think about the importance of maintaining a healthy diet, regular exercise, and other lifestyle modifications while taking Ozempic. Refer to the details in this book with your doctor regarding these lifestyle changes. Implement those changes now - as you start the Ozempic. Not after you have lost the weight.

What Monitoring and Follow-Up Appointments Are Necessary?

Make sure you understand the schedule for blood sugar monitoring and follow-up appointments to assess the effectiveness of the medication. Talk to your doctor about pancreatic and thyroid monitoring.

What Are the Long-Term Effects and Considerations of Taking Ozempic?

Pay attention to news about the long-term implications of using Ozempic, including its effects on diabetes progression and the potential duration of treatment. Discuss how long your doctor feels you should be taking Ozempic, what are the personalized weight loss expectations, and what plan will be implemented once you achieve this goal.

What Should I Do If I Experience Severe Hypoglycemia?

Understand the signs of low blood sugar and how to respond if it occurs while taking Ozempic.

Don't be afraid to talk to your doctor about the cost of Ozempic and alternatives. Many insurance companies are covering these medications. Getting the prescription written by the doctor is only the first step. You need to obtain the medication and without insurance coverage, Ozempic and similar agents can be very expensive.

But in considering these costs, also think about and speak to your doctor about how Ozempic may contribute to cost savings. There are many ways Ozempic can potentially save you money.

Improved blood sugar control: Ozempic can help individuals with type 2 diabetes better manage their blood sugar levels. When blood sugar levels are well-controlled, there may be fewer instances of extremely high or low blood sugar, reducing the need for emergency medical care and associated costs.

Reduction in Medication Costs: For some individuals, Ozempic may replace other diabetes medications that are less effective in controlling blood sugar. This can potentially reduce the need for multiple medications, saving on prescription costs. If you are currently taking medications to manage obesity-related conditions, such as diabetes or high blood pressure, successful weight loss may allow you to reduce or eliminate the need for some of these medications. This can result in savings on prescription drug costs.

Lower Risk of Diabetes-Related Complications: Better blood sugar control with Ozempic can lead to a decreased risk of diabetes-related complications such as kidney disease, heart disease, and vision problems. Avoiding these complications can help save on medical expenses in the long run.

Weight Management: Some people taking Ozempic may experience weight loss or weight management benefits. Maintaining a healthy weight can reduce the risk of obesity-related health conditions, potentially lowering medical costs related to these conditions.

Decreased Food Expenses: Achieving and maintaining a healthy weight often involves making healthier food choices and consuming fewer calories. This can lead to a reduction in grocery bills and dining-out expenses, as you may opt for lower-calorie, more nutritious foods.

Gym Memberships and Weight Loss Programs: Some individuals invest in gym memberships, weight loss programs, or personal trainers to help them lose weight. While these expenses can be worthwhile for some, successful weight loss with Wegovy may reduce the need for these services, resulting in potential savings.

Healthy Lifestyle Choices: When individuals are actively managing their weight and diabetes with medications like Ozempic, they are often more motivated to make healthy lifestyle choices. This may include adopting a balanced diet and regular exercise, which can reduce overall food expenses and prevent dining out at restaurants frequently.

Long-term Savings: Maintaining a healthy weight can have long-term financial benefits. You may experience fewer sick days, increased productivity, and a higher quality of life, which can indirectly lead to improved career prospects and income.

It's important to note that the financial savings associated with Ozempic will vary from person to person, depending on their specific circumstances and the extent to which they were previously struggling with uncontrolled diabetes, weight issues and its associated costs.

13

The Cardiovascular Benefits of Semaglutide Medications

Obesity, a widespread and serious health condition, follows a chronic and often recurring path. It places a significant financial strain on individuals, healthcare systems, and society at large, due to both direct healthcare costs and indirect expenses like loss of productivity. The rising prevalence of obesity, which can lead to multiple health problems and decreased lifespan, is a critical issue for public health.

Individuals with obesity face a heightened risk of cardiovascular diseases (CVD) and cardiometabolic issues, including type 2 diabetes. These risks are heightened due to factors such as insulin resistance, high blood pressure, and abnormal lipid levels. Therefore, the primary objectives in treating obesity are not only to reduce body weight but also to address these cardiometabolic risks. Lifestyle changes, including diet modifications and increased physical activity, are fundamental to weight management. These may be supplemented with medication and, in some cases, bariatric surgery. However, there is limited data on the long-term impact of these treatments on cardiometabolic health.

Semaglutide (Ozempic) a glucagon-like peptide-1 (GLP-1) receptor agonist, has been a game-changer in the management of type 2 diabetes. However, recent studies have shed light on its remarkable cardiovascular benefits, making it a multifaceted medication. This chapter delves into the mechanisms and implications of these cardiovascular benefits.

Semaglutide works by mimicking the action of the incretin hormone GLP-1, which is involved in the regulation of glucose metabolism. It enhances insulin secretion, suppresses glucagon release, and delays gastric emptying. These actions not only aid in glucose control but also contribute to cardiovascular health.

One of the key ways semaglutide benefits cardiovascular health is by influencing risk factors. It has been shown to: Lower systolic and diastolic blood pressure; improve lipid profiles, reduce levels of LDL cholesterol; and aid in weight loss, a significant factor in cardiovascular health.

Beyond risk factor modification, semaglutide has direct effects on the cardiovascular system: Reduction in arterial stiffness, improvement in endothelial function; Possible reduction in atherogenic processes.

Several pivotal trials have highlighted the cardiovascular benefits of semaglutide: The SUSTAIN-6 trial demonstrated a significant reduction in major cardiovascular events (MACE) like heart attack, stroke, and cardiovascular death. Further research is ongoing to understand the long-term impacts and the underlying mechanisms.

The cardiovascular benefits of semaglutide suggest a dual role in both diabetes and cardiovascular risk management. This could lead to changes in prescribing practices, especially for patients with type 2 diabetes at high risk

In high cardiovascular (CV) risk patients with type 2 diabetes, two large clinical studies revealed that semaglutide (administered once a week at 1.0 mg subcutaneously and daily at 14 mg orally) lowered the incidence of major adverse cardiovascular events compared to a placebo. Given that many individuals with obesity do not have diabetes and considering the link between obesity and cardiovascular disease, it's crucial to understand the cardiovascular impact of weight-loss-promoting therapies in those without diabetes.

The STEP 1 and 4 trials, which included participants who were overweight or obese but did not have diabetes, demonstrated that semaglutide significantly reduced body weight compared to placebo. Furthermore, treatment with semaglutide was linked to substantial improvements in some cardiometabolic factors. Analysis of the data from these clinical trials to look at the influence of semaglutide on cardiometabolic risk factors in overweight people without diabetes, examined the effects of combining semaglutide with lifestyle changes, as well as evaluating the consequences of continued versus discontinued semaglutide use under similar conditions. The goals of these analyses were to assess: (a) whether semaglutide improves cardiometabolic risk factors, both overall and in relation to the degree of weight loss; (b) the necessity of ongoing semaglutide therapy to maintain any benefits; and (c) the impact of semaglutide on the risk of atherosclerotic cardiovascular disease and the use of concurrent medications for cardiovascular risk risk factors.

The data from the STEP 1 and 4 trials looked at the impact of semaglutide, administered once weekly subcutaneously at a dose of 2.4 mg and combined with lifestyle modifications, on various cardiometabolic risk factors. These include waist circumference, blood pressure (BP), fasting plasma glucose (FPG), fasting serum insulin, Homeostatic Model Assessment for Insulin Resistance (HOMA-IR), and cholesterol/lipid levels) in adults who are overweight or obese but do not have type 2 diabetes.

The studies observed notable improvements in many of these risk factors with semaglutide use compared to placebo. Additionally, these positive changes led to a reduced necessity for medications that lower blood pressure and lipids in both studies. However, while semaglutide showed non-significant trends toward lowering the predicted 10-year risk of atherosclerotic cardiovascular disease, discontinuing the treatment led to a loss of these cardiometabolic benefits.

Obesity management guidelines suggest aiming for a weight reduction of more than 5% to 15%. In these studies, about 85% of participants achieved a weight loss of at least 5%, with many experiencing even greater reductions. These analyses indicate that larger weight losses were correlated with more significant improvements in cardiometabolic risk factors. The most substantial decreases in these risk factors typically occurred within the first 20 weeks of semaglutide treatment in both studies, paralleling the weight loss trajectory observed with this medication in other studies. However, data also shows that the potential cardiometabolic advantages of semaglutide were not sustained after stopping the medication.

In another study that looked at individuals who are overweight or obese who have established cardiovascular disease (CVD) but do not have diabetes mellitus (DM), a weekly subcutaneous dose of semaglutide was linked to a 20% decrease in major adverse cardiac events over an average period of 33 months. This reduction was notable even amidst widespread use of statins at the same time.

Overall, the latest published studies indicate that patients who received 2.4 mg of semaglutide through weekly subcutaneous injections had a 20% decrease in the combined incidence of cardiovascular death, nonfatal myocardial infarction (heart attack), and nonfatal stroke. Again, the specific extent of these reductions, as well as the length of the treatment and follow-up period are still unknown.

Previous studies focusing on lifestyle changes and pharmacological treatments have not shown a significant impact in lowering the CV risk associated with overweight and obesity.

The mechanisms behind the cardioprotective effects of semaglutide and other GLP-1 agonists are still not completely understood and are probably multifaceted. This is evidenced by the greater reduction in systolic blood pressure and the lower incidence of DM in patients taking semaglutide. This is particularly important considering the high prevalence of prediabetes. It seems that semaglutide could play a broader role in secondary cardiovascular disease prevention among patients without DM who are overweight or obese.

Atherosclerotic cardiovascular disease stands as the leading cause of death and disability among individuals with type 2 diabetes. Patients with type 2 diabetes have been found to experience atherosclerotic heart disease on average 14.6 years earlier, and with a higher risk of mortality, compared to individuals without type 2 diabetes. In the Cardiovascular Outcome Trial, Ozempic when combined with standard care, showed a 26% relative risk reduction in major adverse cardiovascular events after 2 years, with an absolute risk reduction of 2.3% at 109 weeks.

Another clinical trial revealed that administering semaglutide once a week improved health outcomes and quality of life for patients with heart failure and obesity, regardless of their initial health status, compared to a placebo. This extends the insights from an earlier clinical trial, which demonstrated that semaglutide helps patients who have both obesity and heart failure - a condition where the heart muscle becomes rigid, leading to fluid accumulation in the lungs and body — in losing weight. Additionally, it was found to reduce symptoms and boost exercise capacity in these patients.

Another large clinical trial revealed that administering semaglutide once a week improved health outcomes and quality of life for patients with heart failure and obesity, regardless of their initial health status, compared to a placebo.

This extends the insights from an earlier clinical trial, which demonstrated that semaglutide assists patients who have both obesity and heart failure — a condition where the heart muscle becomes rigid, leading to fluid accumulation in the lungs and body — in losing weight. Additionally, it was found to enhance symptoms and boost exercise capacity in these patients.

The researchers discovered that patients on semaglutide, irrespective of their initial health condition, encompassing overall symptoms and quality of life, achieved more significant weight loss and showed more substantial improvements in symptoms related to heart failure, physical constraints, exercise function and blood markers of heart failure and inflammation, when compared to those receiving a placebo.

Finally, semaglutide was linked with enhancements across all areas of patient quality of life and cardiovascular symptoms. While the specific mechanisms by which semaglutide enhances cardiovascular health remain uncertain, it is evident that the medication aids in both the prevention and treatment of cardiovascular disease in patients, regardless of whether they currently have the disease or not.

More research is underway and we anticipate lots of new clinical trial outcomes for GLP-1 agents in terms of cardiovascular disease and other diseases within the next few years.

IV

The Ozempic Diet

14

Diets and Diet Therapy

So we've gone though a lot of the science of hunger and insulin, but now lets look at the world of diets. Weight loss is a vast and diverse industry that encompasses a wide range of products, services, and strategies designed to help individuals lose weight, improve their health, and achieve their fitness goals. It is a multi-billion dollar industry that continues to evolve in response to changing trends, scientific research, and consumer demand.

The weight loss industry has churned out tons of different strategies, over-the-counter supplements, meal replacement shakes, weight loss pills, and herbal remedies. These products often claim to boost metabolism, suppress appetite, or promote fat burning.

Commercial diet programs offer structured meal plans and support for weight loss. Popular examples include Weight Watchers (WW), Jenny Craig, Nutrisystem, and the South Beach Diet.

The industry includes the sale of exercise machines, fitness wearables, and gym memberships. Many individuals turn to exercise as a key component of their weight loss journey. Gyms, fitness studios, and personal trainers provide services to help individuals with weight loss through customized exercise routines, group fitness classes, and one-on-one coaching.

The proliferation of mobile apps and online platforms has made it easier for people to access weight loss tools, track their progress, and receive guidance on diet and exercise.

And then there are medical interventions, such as bariatric surgery, which uses gastric bypass and gastric sleeve procedures, as an intervention for severe obesity. Medical weight loss clinics offer physician-supervised programs that may include prescription medications.

In addition, there are experts in nutrition counseling and dietitians. Registered dietitians and nutritionists provide personalized dietary advice and support to individuals seeking to manage their weight and improve their nutrition. Subscription-based meal delivery services can provide pre-portioned and calorie-controlled meals designed to support weight loss goals.

Behavioral therapists and psychologists offer counseling and therapy to address emotional eating, binge eating, and other psychological factors that can affect weight. Wellness coaches assist individuals in setting and achieving weight loss goals by focusing on overall health and lifestyle factors.

The weight loss industry invests in research to develop new products and approaches based on the latest scientific findings. The industry heavily markets its products and services through advertisements, celebrity endorsements, and social media influencers. Weight loss advertising is one of the leading sources of ads in the world.

Weight loss achieved through various diets, weight loss medications, and over-the-counter supplements can vary widely depending on several factors, including an individual's starting weight, adherence to the program, and overall health. Here is some general information on percentage weight loss achieved with different approaches:

Low-calorie diets typically provide 800 to 1,200 calories per day and can lead to rapid initial weight loss. In clinical studies, individuals on LCDs can achieve weight loss ranging from 5% to 15% of their initial body weight over several months.

Low-carbohydrate diets like the ketogenic diet have been shown to result in significant weight loss. Depending on the duration and adherence, individuals can lose 5% to 10% or more of their initial body weight.

The Mediterranean diet is associated with moderate but sustainable weight loss. On average, participants may lose 5% or more of their initial body weight over several months to a year. This diet has been shown to significantly reduce cardiovascular disease.

Plant-based diets, such as vegetarian and vegan diets, can lead to weight loss of approximately 5% or more of initial body weight, depending on the specific dietary choices and adherence.

But despite calling these all diets, they are really just different ways of eating: Sustainable weight loss often requires long-term changes to diet, physical activity, and lifestyle.

We have discussed some of the other weight loss prescription medications that have come and gone. What are some of the more popular over-the-counter products that are used for weight loss?

Some studies suggest that green tea extract supplements may result in modest weight loss of 2% to 5% of initial body weight over several months. However, results can vary.

The evidence for the effectiveness of Garcinia cambogia in weight loss is mixed. Some studies have shown minimal weight loss, while others have not demonstrated significant effects.

Caffeine supplements may have a mild thermogenic effect and can slightly increase metabolic rate. Weight loss achieved with caffeine supplements is typically minimal (1% to 3% of initial body weight).

Amphetamines, in low doses are also still available over-the-counter and frequently used for short-term weight loss with significant risk for serious side effects.

Obviously, diet plays a crucial role in managing obesity. A well-structured diet plan can help individuals reduce calorie intake, promote weight loss, and improve overall health. Any diet plan for an overweight individual must contain a few key principles and components. The primary goal of a weight loss diet is to create a calorie deficit, where you consume fewer calories than your body burns. If you calculate your daily calorie needs and aim to reduce your calorie intake by a reasonable amount, typically 500 to 1,000 calories per day, you can achieve a gradual and sustainable weight loss of about 1 to 2 pounds per week. But this requires maintaining this caloric reduction.

Although we will discuss in a later chapter, specific dietary changes that you should make when taking Ozempic, we think it is important to go over some general guidelines for lifestyle change to help you be healthy and also contribute to weight loss.

A balanced diet is very important and must include a variety of food groups to ensure that you get essential nutrients. A balanced diet should include:

- Lean Proteins such as poultry, lean meats, fish, tofu, beans, and legumes.
- Whole Grains: whole grains like brown rice, quinoa, whole wheat bread, and oats.
- Fruits and Vegetables: Aim for a colorful variety of fruits and vegetables, which provide vitamins, minerals, and fiber.
- Healthy Fats: Incorporate sources such as avocados, nuts, seeds, and olive oil.
- Dairy or Dairy Alternatives: Opt for low-fat or non-fat options or dairy alternatives like almond or soy milk.
- Limit highly processed foods, sugary beverages, and excessive amounts of added sugars and unhealthy fats.

Be mindful of portion sizes to avoid overeating. Use measuring cups, a kitchen scale, or visual cues to estimate appropriate portion sizes. Avoid eating directly from large packages or containers, as it can lead to over consumption.

Eating regular meals and healthy snacks can help prevent extreme hunger and overeating later in the day. Include protein-rich snacks like Greek yogurt, a handful of nuts, or sliced vegetables with hummus.

Drink plenty of water throughout the day to stay hydrated. Sometimes thirst can be mistaken for hunger. Limit sugary drinks and alcohol, as they can contribute to excess calorie intake.

Practice "Mindful Eating": Pay attention to hunger and fullness cues. Eat slowly and savor your food. Avoid distractions like TV or screens while eating.

Plan your meals and snacks in advance to make healthier choices. Meal planning can help you avoid impulsive, less healthy options.

Incorporate regular physical activity into your routine to boost calorie expenditure and improve overall fitness. Aim for a combination of aerobic exercises (e.g., walking, cycling) and strength training for optimal results.

Focus on adopting dietary habits that can be maintained in the long term. Avoid extreme or restrictive diets that are difficult to sustain. Successful weight loss and obesity management often require a multifaceted approach that includes not only dietary changes but also lifestyle modifications, behavior changes, and ongoing support.

Weight rebound, also known as weight regain, refers to the phenomenon where individuals who have lost weight through diet or drug therapy subsequently regain some or all of the lost weight. Weight rebound is a common challenge and can be frustrating for individuals who have worked hard to achieve weight loss. Several factors contribute to weight rebound after diet or drug therapy:

When you lose weight, especially through calorie restriction or dieting, your body's metabolism often slows down. This is a natural response to conserve energy during periods of reduced calorie intake. As a result, you may require fewer calories to maintain your new lower weight than you did at your previous, higher weight. This can make it easier to regain weight when calorie intake returns to normal.

Hormonal changes can occur with weight loss and impact hunger and satiety signals. Hormones like leptin, which regulates appetite, may decrease after weight loss, making you more prone to overeating. Ghrelin, that hormone that stimulates appetite, may increase after weight loss, potentially increasing hunger and cravings.

Weight rebound can be influenced by psychological factors such as emotional eating, stress, and preoccupation with food. The fear of regaining weight can lead to unhealthy eating patterns or restrictive behaviors, which can backfire and contribute to rebound weight gain.

Unrealistic expectations or goals for weight loss can set individuals up for disappointment and make them more susceptible to rebound weight gain. Sustainable, gradual weight loss is more likely to be maintained than rapid, extreme weight loss.

Successful weight maintenance requires ongoing lifestyle changes, including a balanced diet and regular physical activity. Some individuals may revert to their previous habits once they've achieved their weight loss goals, which can lead to weight regain.

In the context of drug therapy for weight loss, discontinuing the medication can sometimes lead to weight regain if the underlying behaviors and habits that contributed to weight gain are not addressed.

The environment in which you live and work can influence eating behaviors. Access to unhealthy foods, social situations, and stressors can contribute to overeating and weight rebound. Genetics can play a role in an individual's susceptibility to weight rebound. Some people may have a genetic predisposition to regain weight more easily. Weight maintenance can be challenging, and having a support system, including healthcare professionals, family, and friends, can be crucial for long-term success.

To reduce the risk of weight rebound after diet or drug therapy, it's important to set realistic and sustainable weight loss goals. Focus on long-term lifestyle changes, including a balanced diet and regular physical activity. Develop strategies for managing stress and emotional eating. You may also want to seek support from healthcare professionals, such as registered dietitians or therapists.

Remember that maintaining a healthy weight is a lifelong journey, and setbacks are common. It's essential to approach weight management with patience, self-compassion, and a commitment to long-term health and well-being.

15

Sample Meal Plan 1: Balanced Meals

Balanced meals and mindful eating are essential components of a healthy and sustainable approach to nutrition. A balanced meal typically includes a variety of nutrient-rich foods from different food groups, such as lean proteins, whole grains, fruits, vegetables, and healthy fats. This combination ensures that you get a diverse range of essential nutrients, including vitamins, minerals, fiber, and protein, which are crucial for overall well-being. Mindful eating, on the other hand, involves being present and fully engaged in the eating experience. It means savoring each bite, paying attention to hunger and fullness cues, and eating with awareness rather than on autopilot. Practicing mindful eating can help promote a healthier relationship with food, prevent overeating, and enhance satisfaction with meals. By embracing balanced meals and mindful eating, individuals can better support their physical and emotional health while enjoying a diverse and pleasurable diet.

Breakfast:

- Scrambled eggs with spinach and tomatoes.
- Whole-grain toast or a small portion of steel-cut oats.
- A small serving of berries.

Lunch:

- Grilled chicken or tofu salad with mixed greens, cucumbers, and bell peppers.
- Olive oil and balsamic vinaigrette dressing.
- A serving of quinoa or brown rice.

Snack:

- Greek yogurt with a sprinkle of nuts and berries.

Dinner:

- Baked salmon or a plant-based protein like lentils or chickpeas.
- Steamed broccoli and cauliflower.
- A side salad with mixed greens and a light vinaigrette dressing.

Snack (if needed):

- A small apple or carrot sticks with hummus.

16

Sample Meal Plan 2: Low-Carb Approach

Low-carb eating is a dietary approach that restricts the consumption of carbohydrates, primarily found in foods like grains, bread, pasta, and sugary items. Instead, it emphasizes foods rich in protein, healthy fats, and non-starchy vegetables. This approach can help stabilize blood sugar levels, promote weight loss, and improve overall metabolic health, making it popular for managing conditions like type 2 diabetes and obesity. Low-carb diets often include foods like lean meats, fish, nuts, seeds, and leafy greens. However, it's essential to strike a balance and choose complex carbohydrates from sources like whole grains and legumes for fiber and other essential nutrients. Low-carb eating can be effective for some individuals, but it's essential to consult with a healthcare professional before making significant dietary changes to ensure it aligns with individual health goals and needs.

Breakfast:

- Spinach and mushroom omelet with feta cheese.
- Sliced avocado.

Lunch:

- Grilled chicken or tofu with a side of sautéed asparagus and cherry

tomatoes.
- A small mixed greens salad.
- A spinach and arugula salad with grilled shrimp or tempeh.
- An olive oil and lemon dressing.

Snack:

- A handful of mixed nuts.

Dinner:

- Baked fish (e.g., cod, tilapia) with lemon and herbs.
- Roasted Brussels sprouts and cauliflower.
- A side of quinoa or cauliflower rice.

Snack (if needed):

- A small serving of cottage cheese with berries.
- Celery sticks with almond butter.

17

Sample Meal Plan 3: Vegetarian or Vegan Option

Vegetarian and vegan diets are plant-based dietary choices that abstain from or greatly reduce the consumption of animal products. Vegetarians typically exclude meat but may include other animal-derived products like dairy and eggs. Vegans, on the other hand, abstain from all animal products, including dairy, eggs, and honey. These dietary choices are often motivated by ethical, environmental, and health considerations. Vegetarian and vegan diets are rich in fruits, vegetables, whole grains, legumes, nuts, and seeds, which provide essential nutrients like fiber, vitamins, minerals, and antioxidants. These diets have been associated with numerous health benefits, including a reduced risk of chronic diseases such as heart disease, certain cancers, and type 2 diabetes. However, it's important for individuals following these diets to pay attention to getting adequate protein, vitamin B12, iron, and other nutrients that may be less abundant in plant-based foods, and they should consider consulting with a healthcare professional or registered dietitian to ensure their nutritional needs are met.

Breakfast:

- Overnight oats made with almond milk, chia seeds, and topped with sliced bananas and a drizzle of honey (or a vegan sweetener).

- A smoothie with spinach, kale, banana, and almond milk.
- A scoop of protein powder (check for added sugars).

Lunch:

- Lentil and vegetable soup.
- A side salad with mixed greens, cucumbers, and vinaigrette dressing.
- A side of brown rice.

Snack:

- Sliced bell peppers with hummus.
- Cottage cheese with sliced peaches.
- A small serving of unsweetened, non-dairy yogurt with a sprinkle of berries.

Dinner:

- Stir-fried tofu or tempeh with broccoli, bell peppers, and snow peas in a low-sugar teriyaki sauce.
- Brown rice or cauliflower rice.
- Stuffed bell peppers with a mixture of quinoa, black beans, corn, and salsa.
- A side salad with mixed greens and balsamic vinaigrette.

18

Sample Meal Plan 4: Balanced Macronutrients

Balancing macronutrients, including carbohydrates, proteins, and fats, is a fundamental principle of healthy eating. Each macronutrient serves a unique role in the body, and a well-balanced diet ensures that you receive a diverse array of nutrients for optimal health. Carbohydrates provide energy, and they should come from whole grains, fruits, and vegetables for fiber and vitamins. Proteins are essential for muscle repair and overall body function, and sources like lean meats, poultry, fish, legumes, and tofu are great choices. Healthy fats, found in foods like avocados, nuts, seeds, and olive oil, support brain health and aid in nutrient absorption. Balancing these macronutrients in your meals can help regulate blood sugar, maintain energy levels, and keep you feeling satisfied. While the ideal balance varies from person to person, focusing on whole, nutrient-dense foods and portion control is key to achieving a well-rounded and nourishing diet.

Breakfast:

- Scrambled eggs with spinach and tomatoes.
- A small serving of steel-cut oats topped with berries.
- Herbal tea or black coffee (without added sugar).

Lunch:

- Grilled chicken breast or tofu salad with mixed greens, cucumbers, and cherry tomatoes.
- A vinaigrette dressing made with olive oil and vinegar.
- A side of quinoa or brown rice.

Snack:

- Greek yogurt with a sprinkle of cinnamon and a few almonds.

Dinner:

- Baked salmon or a vegetarian lentil stew.
- Steamed broccoli or asparagus.
- A small serving of roasted sweet potatoes.

19

Sample Meal Plan 5: Mediterranean-Inspired

The Mediterranean Diet is a dietary pattern inspired by the traditional eating habits of countries bordering the Mediterranean Sea. It's celebrated for its potential health benefits and delicious, diverse food choices. This diet emphasizes whole, minimally processed foods such as fruits, vegetables, whole grains, legumes, nuts, and seeds. Olive oil is a central source of healthy fats, replacing saturated fats like butter. Lean proteins, particularly fish and poultry, are consumed in moderate amounts, and red meat is limited. Herbs and spices add flavor without excessive salt. The Mediterranean Diet is recognized for its potential to lower the risk of chronic diseases, including heart disease, diabetes, and certain cancers. Its emphasis on plant-based foods, healthy fats, and moderate protein intake provides a well-rounded approach to nutrition, promoting overall health and longevity.

Breakfast:

- Greek yogurt parfait with fresh berries, honey, and a sprinkle of walnuts.

Lunch:

- Hummus and vegetable wrap with whole-grain flatbread.
- A side of tabbouleh salad.

Snack:

- Sliced cucumbers and cherry tomatoes with tzatziki sauce.

Dinner:

- Grilled or baked fish (e.g., tilapia or salmon) with a lemon-dill sauce.
- Roasted mixed vegetables.
- Quinoa or bulgur as a side.

20

Tailored Diets for Ozempic Users

Balancing macronutrients in the diet involves ensuring that you consume an appropriate and well-proportioned amount of the three primary macronutrients: carbohydrates, proteins, and fats. Achieving this balance can contribute to overall health, help manage weight, and support various bodily functions. Here's how to balance macronutrients in your diet:

Carbohydrates:
   Carbohydrates are a primary source of energy for the body. Focus on complex carbohydrates like whole grains (e.g., brown rice, quinoa, oats), legumes (e.g., beans, lentils), and starchy vegetables (e.g., sweet potatoes). Limit simple carbohydrates, such as sugars and refined grains (e.g., white bread, sugary cereals, pastries).

Proteins:
   Proteins are essential for tissue repair, immune function, and muscle growth. Include lean protein sources like poultry, fish, tofu, beans, legumes, low-fat dairy, and lean cuts of meat. Balance protein intake throughout the day to support muscle maintenance and overall satiety.

Fats:
   Healthy fats are important for cell function, nutrient absorption, and

hormone production. Include sources of unsaturated fats like avocados, nuts, seeds, and olive oil. Limit saturated fats found in fatty meats, full-fat dairy, and processed foods. Minimize trans fats, often found in partially hydrogenated oils and many processed and fried foods.

Portion Control:

Pay attention to portion sizes to avoid overeating and maintain a healthy weight.Use measuring cups, food scales, or portion control containers if needed. Be mindful of calorie intake relative to your activity level and goals.

Dietary Fiber:

Include high-fiber foods like fruits, vegetables, whole grains, and legumes in your diet. Fiber aids in digestion helps control blood sugar levels, and promotes satiety.

Meal Timing and Frequency:

Distribute macronutrients evenly throughout the day to maintain steady energy levels and prevent extreme fluctuations in blood sugar. Consider smaller, balanced meals and snacks at regular intervals.

Hydration:

Adequate hydration is crucial for overall health and can support balanced nutrition. Water should be the primary beverage of choice. Limit sugary drinks and excessive caffeine intake.

Individualized Needs:

Tailor your macronutrient balance to your individual health goals, activity level, age, and any specific dietary requirements or restrictions. Seek guidance from a registered dietitian or healthcare provider for personalized recommendations.

Balancing macronutrients in your diet is not a one-size-fits-all approach; it should be adjusted based on individual factors. Regular monitoring of your dietary choices, physical activity, and health status can help you maintain a balanced diet that supports your overall well-being.

Complex Carbohydrates:
Prioritize complex carbohydrates like whole grains, legumes, and vegetables over simple carbohydrates and refined sugars. Complex carbs have a lower impact on blood sugar.

Fiber-Rich Foods:
Include foods high in dietary fiber, such as fruits, vegetables, whole grains, and legumes. Fiber helps control blood sugar levels and promotes satiety.

Lean Proteins:
Opt for lean protein sources like poultry, fish, tofu, beans, and low-fat dairy products. Protein can help stabilize blood sugar and keep you feeling full.

Healthy Fats:
Incorporate sources of healthy fats, such as avocados, nuts, seeds, and olive oil, while limiting saturated and trans fats.

Portion Control:
Be mindful of portion sizes to avoid overeating. Measuring food or using portion-control containers can be helpful.

Regular Meals
Try to eat at consistent times each day and include healthy snacks if needed to prevent extreme fluctuations in blood sugar.

Low-Glycemic Foods
Choose foods with a low glycemic index (GI) to help stabilize blood sugar levels. Examples include quinoa, sweet potatoes, and most non-starchy vegetables.

Limit Added Sugars

Minimize or eliminate sugary snacks, candies, and sugary beverages.

Hydration

Stay well-hydrated with water and unsweetened beverages. Limit sugary drinks.

Alcohol in Moderation

If you consume alcohol, do so in moderation, and consider its impact on blood sugar levels.

Regular Monitoring

Monitor blood sugar levels as recommended by your healthcare provider and adjust your diet accordingly.

Consult a Dietitian

Work with a registered dietitian to create a personalized meal plan tailored to your specific needs, taking into account your health goals, lifestyle, and any dietary restrictions.

Remember that Ozempic should be used as part of a comprehensive diabetes management plan. Your healthcare provider or dietitian can provide specific dietary recommendations and help you make necessary adjustments to your diet based on your individual health status and goals

Alcohol consumption can have different effects on individuals with prediabetes and diabetes. While moderate alcohol consumption may have certain benefits, it's essential for individuals with these conditions to be aware of how alcohol can impact blood sugar levels and overall health. Here's some guidance for alcohol consumption for individuals with prediabetes and diabetes:

Prediabetes is a condition in which blood sugar levels are higher than normal but not yet in the diabetic range. It is an important time to make lifestyle changes to prevent the progression to type 2 diabetes. If you choose to consume alcohol, it's generally advisable to do so in moderation. Moderate alcohol consumption for men is typically defined as up to two drinks per day, while for women, it's up to one drink per day.

Be mindful of the carbohydrate content of alcoholic beverages, as they can affect blood sugar levels.Regularly monitor your blood sugar levels to understand how alcohol affects you personally.

Alcohol can lead to hypoglycemia (low blood sugar) in individuals with type 1 diabetes, particularly if consumed on an empty stomach or in excess. It's essential to consume alcohol in moderation and to eat a balanced meal or snack with carbohydrates when drinking.Keep track of your blood sugar levels and have a plan to treat hypoglycemia if it occurs.

Individuals with type 2 diabetes should also consume alcohol in moderation. Alcohol can lead to both hypoglycemia and hyperglycemia (high blood sugar) depending on factors like the type of alcohol, the quantity consumed, and individual tolerance. Test your blood sugar before and after drinking to understand its impact on your levels. Avoid excessive drinking, which can lead to poor blood sugar control, liver problems, and other health complications.

For all people, both diabetic and non diabetic, choose alcoholic beverages that are lower in sugar and carbohydrates when possible. For example, dry wines or light beers typically have fewer carbohydrates than sugary cocktails. Avoid binge drinking, as it can have serious health consequences and negatively affect blood sugar control. And alcohol can interact with some diabetes medications, so consult with your healthcare provider to understand any potential interactions and receive personalized guidance.

Some individuals with diabetes, particularly those with certain complica-tions or other medical conditions, may be advised to avoid alcohol entirely. Always follow your healthcare provider's recommendations. Alcohol can impair judgment and increase the risk of hypoglycemia. Make sure someone is aware of your diabetes and knows how to help in case of an emergency when you are drinking.

In summary, while moderate alcohol consumption may be acceptable for some individuals with prediabetes and diabetes, it's crucial to be cautious and monitor its effects on blood sugar levels.

Low glycemic foods are those that have a relatively mild impact on blood sugar levels when consumed, as they are digested and absorbed more slowly. These foods have a lower glycemic index (GI) compared to high-GI foods, which can cause rapid spikes and crashes in blood sugar. Incorporating low-GI foods into your diet can help stabilize blood sugar levels and provide sustained energy. Some low-glycemic foods include:

Non-Starchy Vegetables:
leafy greens (spinach, kale, arugula), broccoli, cauliflower, zucchini, bell peppers, cucumber, tomatoes

Legumes and Pulses:
lentils, chickpeas, kidney beans, black beans, pinto beans

Whole Grains:
oats (steel-cut or rolled), quinoa, barley, bulgur, whole wheat pasta, brown rice

Fruits:
berries (strawberries, blueberries, raspberries), cherries, apples, pears, oranges, grapefruit

Dairy and Dairy Alternatives:
greek yogurt (plain, unsweetened), milk (whole or low-fat), soy milk (unsweetened), almond milk (unsweetened), cottage cheese

Nuts and Seeds:
almonds, walnuts, peanuts, chia seeds, flaxseeds, pumpkin seeds

Proteins:
lean meats (chicken, turkey, lean cuts of beef), fish (salmon, trout, mackerel), tofu and tempeh. eggs

Sweeteners (in moderation):

stevia, erythritol, monk fruit extract

Vegetable Oils:

olive oil, canola oil, avocado oil

Herbs and Spices:

Most herbs and spices, such as basil, oregano, cinnamon, and turmeric, have negligible effects on blood sugar and can be used to add flavor to dishes without increasing the glycemic index. It's important to note that the glycemic index can vary based on factors like ripeness, preparation, and cooking methods.

The American Diabetes Association (ADA) provides dietary guidelines and recommendations for people with diabetes. These guidelines are designed to help individuals manage their blood sugar levels, achieve and maintain a healthy weight, and reduce the risk of diabetes-related complications. The ADA recognizes that there isn't a one-size-fits-all approach to diabetes nutrition, so they offer different eating patterns to accommodate various preferences and needs.

ADA diets often focus on carbohydrate counting, as carbohydrates have the most significant impact on blood sugar levels. Individuals with diabetes are encouraged to monitor their carbohydrate intake, which includes tracking the number of carbohydrate servings consumed in each meal and snack. This approach allows for flexibility in food choices, as long as the total carbohydrate intake is managed to control blood sugar.

The ADA promotes the "Create Your Plate" method, which divides a standard dinner plate into specific portions for different food groups: Half the plate is filled with non-starchy vegetables (e.g., broccoli, spinach).One-quarter of the plate contains lean protein sources (e.g., chicken, fish). One-quarter of the plate is reserved for grains or starchy foods (e.g., rice, pasta). A small serving of fruit and a serving of dairy or dairy alternatives (e.g., low-fat yogurt) may also be included.

While ADA diets do not strictly emphasize the glycemic index of foods, they do consider it when making dietary recommendations. Foods with a lower GI are preferred because they have a milder impact on blood sugar levels.

ADA guidelines often recommend spreading meals and snacks throughout the day to help manage blood sugar levels and prevent extreme fluctuations. Regular meal timing and portion control are emphasized.

ADA diets are tailored to individual needs and preferences. They take into account factors such as age, activity level, medication, and personal food choices. The ADA recognizes that there is no one "diabetes diet" and encourages individuals to work with healthcare providers and registered dietitians to create a personalized nutrition plan.

Regular blood sugar monitoring is essential to assess how dietary choices affect blood glucose levels. Diabetes education, often provided by certified diabetes educators, helps individuals understand the principles of ADA diets and how to make healthy food choices.

ADA diets promote overall health and encourage individuals to choose nutrient-dense foods, limit added sugars, reduce saturated and trans fats, and control portion sizes.It's important to note that ADA diets are just one approach to diabetes nutrition, and they may be adapted to suit individual needs and preferences. Some people with diabetes may also follow other dietary patterns, such as low-carb diets or Mediterranean-style diets, under the guidance of their healthcare team.

21

Special Diet Recommendations to Limit Side Effects

Considering the role of incretins in digestion, it's logical that medications like Ozempic, which modulate the incretin system, can lead to gastrointestinal issues like nausea, vomiting, and diarrhea. Ozempic can induce a sense of fullness by signaling to your brain that you're satiated and by prolonging the presence of food in your stomach, potentially causing nausea when you attempt to eat while taking it.

Fortunately, for most individuals, the nausea is typically mild to moderate and tends to subside as your body adapts to the medication. In the meantime, there are some strategies to alleviate nausea while on Ozempic:

Avoid certain foods that can worsen nausea with Ozempic, such as doughnuts, burgers, fried foods, chips, sausage, canned or processed foods, and other salty or spicy options. Instead, opt for low-fat, bland foods with high water content, like crackers, toast, English muffins, baked chicken, baked fish, potatoes, rice, soup, chicken broth, carrots, fruit without the skin, fruit popsicles, and yogurt.

Change your eating habits by consuming smaller portions more frequently. Eat slowly and savor your meal, stopping when you feel full. Avoid lying down immediately after eating, and refrain from eating right before bedtime.

Choose ice-cold, clear fluids and sip them slowly to stay well-hydrated without overfilling your stomach. Drinking straight from a glass is preferable to using a straw. Consider options like water, herbal tea, and ginger-based beverages, which can help alleviate nausea.

If you're aware of specific triggers for your nausea, such as motion sickness, strong smells, or stress, try to avoid them.

After eating, take a short walk outdoors or engage in light exercise to help settle your stomach. Avoid vigorous activity immediately after a meal.

Vomiting is another potential side effect when using Ozempic, although it's less common than nausea. The likelihood of vomiting varies depending on the dosage and can range from 5% to 9% of individuals taking Ozempic for type 2 diabetes. Vomiting tends to be more prevalent when starting Ozempic or when adjusting the dosage. Higher doses of semaglutide, particularly when used for weight loss, may also increase the likelihood of vomiting. Vomiting can lead to dehydration, so it's crucial to rehydrate by drinking plenty of water if you experience it.

If you encounter severe abdominal pain, possibly accompanied by vomiting, and if this pain radiates to your back, it's essential to promptly contact your healthcare provider. This could be indicative of pancreatitis, a severe inflammation of the pancreas.

Diarrhea is another common side effect of Ozempic, affecting approximately 8% to 9% of individuals using it for type 2 diabetes and 31% of those taking the higher 2.4 mg dose for weight management. Like nausea and vomiting, it is most common when adjusting the Ozempic dosage and usually subsides as your body adapts to the medication. If you experience diarrhea while taking Ozempic, stay hydrated by consuming ample fluids, as diarrhea can lead to dehydration.

Some individuals may encounter mild to moderate stomach discomfort, pain, or bloating when using Ozempic. This side effect affects fewer than one in ten Ozempic users. For relief, consider taking a warm bath or using a heating pad.

However, severe stomach pain, especially if it persists and may or may not be accompanied by vomiting, could indicate a more serious issue, such as pancreatitis. In such cases, it's crucial to contact your healthcare provider promptly and follow their medical guidance.

Around 5% of individuals may experience constipation as a side effect of Ozempic. While less common than other gastrointestinal side effects, constipation can last longer. In some instances, individuals taking a high dose of semaglutide for weight loss reported constipation for nearly a month, compared to only a few days of nausea, vomiting, or diarrhea.

Fortunately, many strategies for relieving constipation can also benefit blood sugar control and weight management, both of which Ozempic can help with. Regular exercise, in particular, can alleviate constipation and offer added advantages for those managing type 2 diabetes or weight.

Additionally, some people taking Ozempic may experience additional gastrointestinal side effects, such as mild burping, flatulence, and acid reflux. Eating more slowly can help mitigate these side effects since burping and flatulence can occur when you swallow excess air, which is more likely to happen when eating too quickly.

Drinking plenty of water and limiting carbonated beverages can also be beneficial. Several of the foods that should be avoided while taking Ozempic can contribute to acid reflux, including high-fat foods, carbonated drinks, and spicy, salty, or fried foods. Reducing your intake of these foods can be advantageous for managing diabetes and minimizing the risk of heartburn.

While it's important for people with type 2 diabetes to consume foods with the recommended minimum daily fiber intake, excessive fiber intake can lead to flatulence. If persistent flatulence is an issue, consult your healthcare provider or a nutritionist for guidance on adjusting your diet to obtain sufficient fiber without needing supplements.

Pancreatitis, a rare but serious side effect of Ozempic, refers to severe inflammation of the pancreas. If you experience persistent, severe stomach pain, discontinue the use of Ozempic and contact your healthcare provider immediately. This pain may radiate to your back, and vomiting may or may not accompany it. If pancreatitis is confirmed by your healthcare provider, they will address the pain and might suggest alternative diabetes or weight loss medications in place of Ozempic.

Diabetic retinopathy is a term used to describe changes in vision that may arise as a complication of type 2 diabetes. In clinical trials, individuals taking Ozempic faced a higher likelihood of experiencing diabetic retinopathy complications, especially if they had a history of this condition.

It is worth noting that diabetic retinopathy can sometimes temporarily worsen when there is a sudden improvement in blood glucose levels, a situation that can occur with the use of Ozempic. Signs of diabetic retinopathy may include blurred vision, the perception of floaters, and partial or complete vision loss.

Should you notice any alterations in your vision while taking Ozempic, it is crucial to inform your healthcare provider. Additionally, be sure to disclose any history of diabetic retinopathy before commencing Ozempic therapy.

While rare, individuals who take blood sugar-lowering medications like insulin or sulfonylureas may face an elevated risk of experiencing hypoglycemia (low blood sugar) when using Ozempic. If you are concurrently taking insulin or sulfonylureas, your healthcare provider may adjust the dosage of these drugs to minimize the risk of hypoglycemia.

In case you observe signs of low blood sugar, promptly contact your healthcare provider. Symptoms of hypoglycemia encompass dizziness, sweating, confusion, drowsiness, headache, blurred vision, slurred speech, shakiness, palpitations, hunger, muscle weakness, jitteriness, anxiety, irritability, or mood swings.

The use of GLP-1 receptor agonists, including Ozempic, can potentially worsen kidney function or result in kidney injury, even in individuals without pre-existing chronic kidney disease. A noticeable sign of acute kidney injury is a decrease in urine output, accompanied by potential fatigue or swelling.

Kidney problems are more likely in those experiencing side effects like nausea, vomiting, diarrhea, and dehydration, which can occur with Ozempic use. If such side effects arise while taking Ozempic, it's essential to ensure proper hydration by drinking ample fluids.

If you have a history of kidney issues, it's vital to inform your healthcare provider before starting Ozempic to enable them to exercise caution when adjusting your dosage.

While exceedingly rare, less than 1% of individuals may encounter an uncommon injection site reaction, such as a rash or itching, at the site of Ozempic injection. However, some individuals may have allergies to semaglutide or the inactive ingredients in Ozempic, which can trigger a severe allergic reaction.

Semaglutide is the primary active ingredient in Ozempic, and the formulation includes other inactive ingredients like disodium phosphate dihydrate, propylene glycol, and phenol, which could potentially elicit reactions.

Gallbladder issues, specifically cholelithiasis (gallstones), are a rare but conceivable side effect when using Ozempic or Wegovy. These problems affect fewer than 3% of individuals taking Ozempic for weight loss or type 2 diabetes. Signs of gallbladder issues may involve sharp and persistent abdominal pain, possibly accompanied by nausea, vomiting, or sweating.

In certain cases, gallstones may be asymptomatic and not necessitate treatment, while more severe complications may require surgical removal of the gallbladder. Adopting a low-fat diet, engaging in regular exercise, and achieving weight loss can help prevent gallstones. It is essential to inform your healthcare provider if you have a history of gallbladder disease before initiating Ozempic.

Lastly, a very small number of individuals may experience dysgeusia when using Ozempic. Dysgeusia is a taste disorder characterized by altered taste perceptions, such as a bitter or metallic taste in foods.

22

General Ozempic Diet Rules

The Ozempic diet is multifaceted. It takes knowledge and strategic implementation for it to be successful. Allow yourself grace as you try it out day-by-day, meal-by-meal. Once you master our recommended go-to meals, snacks, and Ozempic recipes, you'll never be at a loss for what to eat. You will feel satisfied and more importantly feel great satisfaction, even joy!, while eating a variety of foods and still losing weight.

Ozempic typically causes 15% body weight loss

Here are the key elements to this diet:

- Low in calories
- Low in volume
- Low in sugar
- Low in carbohydrates
- Low acidic
- High in protein
- Easy to digest
- Helps prevent nausea

You can try the following meal ideas and guidelines. However, please keep in mind that individual tolerance to foods can vary, so it's essential to listen to your body and adjust as needed.

General Guidelines:

- Small and Frequent Meals: Instead of three large meals, opt for smaller, more frequent meals throughout the day. This can help prevent overloading your stomach.
- Hydration: Stay well-hydrated with water or herbal teas, but avoid very cold or very hot beverages, as extreme temperatures can trigger nausea.
- Avoid Strong Odors: Strong-smelling foods can sometimes exacerbate nausea. Opt for bland or mild-smelling options.
- Ginger: Ginger is known for its anti-nausea properties. Consider incorporating ginger tea or ginger-flavored foods into your diet.
- Chew Slowly: Chew your food slowly and thoroughly to aid digestion.

Here are some helpful meal suggestions:

Breakfast Options:

- Plain Greek yogurt and berries: Greek yogurt is high in protein and easy to digest. Add a small amount of low-glycemic berries for sweetness
- Oatmeal with almond butter and berries: Cooked oats are gentle on the stomach. Top with a tablespoon of almond butter for protein and some fresh berries or a dash of maple syrup
- Scrambled Eggs with Spinach: Scrambled eggs provide high-quality protein. Cook with spinach for added nutrients without increasing volume.

Lunch and Dinner Options:

- Chicken or Tofu Soup: Clear chicken or vegetable broth-based soups are soothing. Include small pieces of chicken or tofu for protein.
- Baked or Grilled Salmon with Steamed Vegetables: Salmon is a great source of protein and healthy fats. Steam some easy-to-digest vegetables like zucchini, carrots, or spinach.
- Mashed Potatoes with Lean Ground Turkey: Make mashed potatoes with a small amount of butter or olive oil. Top with lean ground turkey for protein.
- Quinoa Salad with Cucumber and Chickpeas: Quinoa is easy to digest and high in protein. Add cucumber, chickpeas, and a light vinaigrette for flavor.

Snack Options:

- Cottage Cheese with dark chocolate nibs: Cottage cheese is rich in protein. 70% percent dark chocolate nibs can add a touch of sweetness and crunch without excess sugar
- Rice Cakes with Almond Butter: Rice cakes are gentle on the stomach. Spread a thin layer of almonds for protein.
- Banana and Almonds: Bananas are easy on the stomach and provide some natural sugars. Almonds offer protein and healthy fats.

Beverages:

- Herbal Teas: Ginger, peppermint, or chamomile tea can help soothe the stomach.
- Water with Lemon: Staying hydrated is crucial. Adding lemon can provide a touch of flavor.

Remember to eat small, frequent meals throughout the day to avoid over-whelming your stomach. Additionally, avoid spicy, greasy, and heavily processed foods, as they can exacerbate nausea and digestive discomfort.

Listen to your body and adjust portion sizes and ingredients based on your individual tolerance. If nausea persists or worsens, consult a healthcare professional for further guidance.

Sample Daily Plan:

Breakfast:

- Greek Yogurt: Low in sugar and high in protein.
- Berries: A mild, easy-to-digest, low-glycemic fruit. High in antioxidants.
- Ginger Tea: A warm cup of ginger tea can help settle your stomach.

Snack:

- Crackers: Choose plain, saltine, or whole-grain crackers, which are easy on the stomach. Seed crackers are highly recommended.
- Cottage Cheese: High in protein and relatively easy to digest.

Lunch:

- Chicken Soup: A mild, low-fat, and easy-to-digest option. Use lean chicken breast and add some rice rice or chickpea noodles if desired.
- Steamed Vegetables: Choose well-cooked and easy-to-digest options like carrots, zucchini, or green beans.
- Herbal Tea: A soothing beverage that can help with nausea.

Snack:

- Applesauce: Unsweetened applesauce is easy on the stomach and low in sugar.
- Almonds: A small handful of almonds for some protein and healthy fats.

Dinner:

- Baked or Grilled Fish: Salmon or tilapia are good choices. They're high in protein and generally easy to digest.
- Mashed Sweet or Purple Potatoes: Creamy mashed potatoes can be easy on the stomach. Purple potatoes are a recommended "Blue Zone" staple.
- Steamed Spinach: A mild leafy green that's rich in nutrients.
- Peppermint Tea: Peppermint can also help soothe the stomach.

Bedtime Snack (if needed):

- Low-fat Cottage Cheese: A small serving can provide sustained protein throughout the night without overloading your stomach.

Remember to customize this plan according to your individual preferences and sensitivities. It's crucial to consult with a healthcare professional, especially if your nausea persists or worsens, as it could be a sign of an underlying medical condition. They can provide tailored advice and address any specific dietary restrictions you may have.

23

Week Long Ozempic Meal Plan

Here is a week long structured meal plan for someone taking Ozempic. Of course, the recommendations may be modified based upon your personal preferences and any side effects you may have while taking the medication:

This plan emphasizes balanced meals with complex carbohydrates, fiber, lean proteins, and healthy fats. Portion control is essential. Here's the week-long plan:

Day 1:

- Breakfast: Greek yogurt with berries and a sprinkle of chia seeds.
- Snack: Sliced cucumber and hummus.
- Lunch: Grilled chicken breast with mixed greens, cherry tomatoes, and vinaigrette dressing.
- Snack: Almonds or walnuts.
- Dinner: Baked salmon with quinoa and steamed broccoli.

Day 2:

- Breakfast: Oatmeal topped with sliced banana and a teaspoon of almond butter.
- Snack: Carrot and celery sticks with guacamole.

- Lunch: Lentil and vegetable soup with a side salad.
- Snack: Greek yogurt or cottage cheese with a few apple slices.
- Dinner: Stir-fried tofu with mixed vegetables and brown rice.

Day 3:

- Breakfast: Scrambled eggs with spinach and a small serving of whole-grain toast.
- Snack: Sliced bell peppers with hummus.
- Lunch: Quinoa salad with chickpeas, cucumber, and feta cheese.
- Snack: Mixed berries.
- Dinner: Grilled shrimp with roasted sweet potatoes and steamed asparagus.

Day 4:

- Breakfast: Smoothie with spinach, frozen berries, Greek yogurt, and a teaspoon of flaxseed.
- Snack: A small handful of mixed nuts.
- Lunch: Turkey and avocado wrap with whole-grain tortilla.
- Snack: Sliced apple with a teaspoon of peanut butter.
- Dinner: Baked chicken breast with quinoa and roasted Brussels sprouts.

Day 5:

- Breakfast: Cottage cheese with sliced peaches and a drizzle of honey.
- Snack: Sliced cucumber and cherry tomatoes.
- Lunch: Mixed bean salad with avocado, corn, and cilantro.
- Snack: A hard-boiled egg.
- Dinner: Grilled tofu with brown rice and steamed green beans.

Day 6:

- Breakfast: Whole-grain waffles topped with plain yogurt and mixed berries.
- Snack: Celery sticks with almond butter.
- Lunch: Spinach and feta-stuffed chicken breast with a side of roasted cauliflower.
- Snack: A handful of grapes.
- Dinner: Baked cod with quinoa and sautéed spinach.

Day 7:

- Breakfast: Vegetable omelet with a side of sliced tomatoes.
- Snack: Mixed nuts or seeds.
- Lunch: Lentil and vegetable stir-fry with a small serving of brown rice.
- Snack: Sliced pear with cottage cheese.
- Dinner: Grilled lean steak with sweet potato fries and steamed broccoli.

Remember to stay hydrated by drinking plenty of water throughout the day, and consider consulting a healthcare professional or registered dietitian for personalized guidance tailored to your specific insulin resistance needs.

V

Eating On Ozempic

24

Recipes

Here we introduce a collection of recipes thoughtfully crafted to support patients on their Ozempic journey, where controlling blood sugar and achieving weight loss are paramount goals. These recipes not only align with the Ozempic regimen but also serve as inspiring examples for those seeking delicious, health-conscious meals. Each dish is designed to strike a perfect balance between flavor and nutrition, incorporating ingredients that aid in blood sugar management while promoting satiety. These culinary creations are a testament to how mindful cooking can be both therapeutic and delectable, showcasing the synergy between Ozempic and a wholesome, fulfilling diet.

25

The O-melet

If you're looking for a healthy omelet recipe that's suitable for someone with diabetes or you just want to make a delicious omelet, here's a basic recipe you can follow:

```
Ingredients:
2 large eggs
2 tablespoons of water
Salt and pepper to taste
Cooking spray or a small amount of oil (olive oil or canola oil
are good choices)
1/4 cup of diced vegetables (bell peppers, onions, tomatoes,
spinach, mushrooms, etc.)
1/4 cup of diced lean protein (cooked chicken, turkey, ham, or
tofu)
1/4 cup of shredded cheese (optional, and be mindful of the
portion)
```

Instructions:

- In a bowl, whisk the eggs and water together until well beaten. Season with a pinch of salt and a dash of pepper.

- Heat a non-stick skillet over medium-high heat and lightly coat it with cooking spray or a small amount of oil.
- Add the diced vegetables to the skillet and sauté them until they become tender, usually for 2-3 minutes.
- Pour the beaten egg mixture over the sautéed vegetables in the skillet. Allow it to cook without stirring for a minute or so until the edges start to set.
- Gently lift the edges of the omelet with a spatula to let the uncooked eggs flow underneath. Continue cooking until the omelet is mostly set but still slightly runny on top.
- Add the diced protein of your choice (chicken, turkey, ham, or tofu) and sprinkle shredded cheese, if desired, on one half of the omelet.
- Carefully fold the other half of the omelet over the filling to create a half-moon shape.
- Cook for another minute or so until the cheese is melted, and the omelet is cooked through but not browned.
- Slide the omelet onto a plate and serve hot. You can garnish it with fresh herbs or salsa if you like.

26

The O-La-La Muffin

If you're looking for a recipe for a muffin that is suitable for someone with type 2 diabetes or is mindful of their blood sugar levels, you may want to consider making a low-carb or diabetic-friendly muffin. Here's a basic recipe for a low-carb almond flour muffin that you can try:

```
Ingredients:

1 1/2 cups almond flour
1/4 cup coconut flour
1/4 cup granulated sugar substitute (e.g., erythritol or stevia)
1 tsp baking powder
1/4 tsp salt 3 large eggs
1/4 cup melted butter or coconut oil
1/4 cup unsweetened almond milk
1 tsp vanilla extract
Optional add-ins: chopped nuts, berries, or sugar-free chocolate
chips
```

Instructions:

- Preheat your oven to 350°F (175°C) and line a muffin tin with paper liners.

- In a mixing bowl, whisk together the almond flour, coconut flour, sugar substitute, baking powder, and salt.
- In another bowl, beat the eggs and then mix in the melted butter or coconut oil, almond milk, and vanilla extract.
- Combine the wet and dry ingredients, stirring until well combined. If you're using any optional add-ins, fold them into the batter.
- Divide the batter evenly among the muffin cups.
- Bake in the preheated oven for 18-20 minutes or until a toothpick inserted into the center of a muffin comes out clean.
- Allow the muffins to cool in the tin for a few minutes, then transfer them to a wire rack to cool completely.

27

Smooth Into Slim

```
Ingredients:
1/2 cup unsweetened almond milk (or another low-sugar milk
alternative)
1/2 cup Greek yogurt (unsweetened)
1/2 cup frozen mixed berries (blueberries, strawberries,
raspberries)
1/2 small banana (optional for added sweetness, but use in
moderation)
1 tablespoon chia seeds (optional for added fiber and omega-3s)
1/2 teaspoon cinnamon (for flavor and potential blood sugar
regulation)
Ice cubes (optional for thickness)
```

Instructions:

- Add the almond milk and Greek yogurt to your blender.
- Add the frozen mixed berries and banana (if using).
- Sprinkle in the chia seeds and cinnamon.
- If you prefer a thicker smoothie, add a handful of ice cubes.
- Blend until smooth. If it's too thick, you can add more almond milk to

reach your desired consistency.

· Taste and adjust sweetness if necessary. If needed, you can add a sugar substitute like Stevia or a small amount of honey (use sparingly).

This smoothie is designed to be lower in added sugars, but individual responses to foods can vary.

28

t-O-asts

These toast recipes are easy on the digestive system, as they use whole-grain, low-carb or gluten-free bread. They also include healthy fats and low-glycemic index toppings. Toasts provide a good balance of nutrients and are relatively low in calories. Adjust the portion sizes according to your dietary needs and preferences.

Avocado and Tomato Toast:

```
Ingredients:
1 slice of whole-grain or low-carb bread (look for bread with a
low glycemic index)
1/2 ripe avocado, mashed
1 small tomato, sliced
Salt and pepper to taste
Optional: a sprinkle of chia seeds or flaxseeds for added fiber
```

Instructions:

- Toast the bread until it's lightly crispy.
- Spread the mashed avocado evenly on the toast.
- Top with sliced tomatoes and season with salt and pepper.

· Optional: sprinkle with chia or flaxseeds for extra nutrition.

Almond Butter and Banana Toast:

```
Ingredients
1 slice of whole-grain or low-carb bread
1 tablespoon almond butter (unsweetened)
1/2 banana, sliced
A dash of cinnamon (optional)
Instructions:
Toast the bread until it's lightly crispy.
```

Instructions:

· Spread the almond butter on the toast.
· Top with banana slices and a dash of cinnamon for extra flavo

Cottage Cheese and Berries Toast:

```
Ingredients
1 slice of whole-grain or low-carb bread
1/2 cup low-fat cottage cheese
1/2 cup mixed berries (e.g., strawberries, blueberries,
raspberries)
A drizzle of honey (optional)
```

Instructions:

· Toast the bread until it's lightly crispy.
· Spread a layer of cottage cheese on the toast.
· Top with mixed berries.
· Optionally, drizzle with a small amount of honey for added sweetness.

29

The Skinny Sandwich

This sandwich is rich in fiber from the whole-grain bread and vegetables, contains lean protein from the grilled chicken, and includes healthy fats from the avocado. It's a balanced and diabetes-friendly option

```
Ingredients:
For the Grilled Chicken:
2 boneless, skinless chicken breasts
1 tablespoon olive oil
1 teaspoon garlic powder
1 teaspoon paprika
Salt and pepper to taste

For the Sandwich:
4 slices of whole-grain bread (choose bread with high fiber
content)
1 cup mixed fresh vegetables (e.g., lettuce, tomato slices,
cucumber, bell peppers)
1/2 avocado, sliced
1/4 red onion, thinly sliced
2 tablespoons hummus (low-sugar if available)
Optional: Dijon mustard or low-sugar dressing for added flavor
```

·

Instructions:

Grilled Chicken:

- Preheat your grill or a grill pan over medium-high heat.
- In a bowl, mix together olive oil, garlic powder, paprika, salt, and pepper.
- Brush the chicken breasts with the olive oil mixture.
- Grill the chicken for about 6-8 minutes per side or until cooked through, with no pink in the center.
- Remove the chicken from the grill and let it rest for a few minutes before slicing it into thin strips.
- ·

Assembling the Sandwich:

- Toast the whole-grain bread slices [easier to digest]
- On one slice of bread, spread a thin layer of hummus.
- Layer the grilled chicken slices on top of the hummus.
- Add the mixed fresh vegetables, avocado slices, and red onion on top of the chicken.
- Optionally, add a small amount of Dijon mustard or low-sugar dressing for extra flavor.
- Top the sandwich with the second slice of bread.
- Cut the sandwich in half and serve.

30

Sip to Slim Soup

```
Ingredients:
1 tablespoon olive oil
1 small onion, chopped
2 cloves garlic, minced
1 cup lean ground turkey
2 cups low-sodium chicken or vegetable broth
1 cup water
1 can (15 ounces) diced tomatoes (no added sugar)
1 cup chopped broccoli florets
1 cup chopped cauliflower florets
1 cup chopped spinach or kale
1/2 cup chopped bell peppers (red, green, or yellow)
1/2 teaspoon dried thyme
1/2 teaspoon dried rosemary
Salt and pepper to taste
1 cup cooked and drained kidney beans or chickpeas (optional for
added protein)
Fresh parsley for garnish (optional)
```

Instructions:

- In a large pot, heat the olive oil over medium heat. Add the chopped onion and minced garlic, and sauté until they become fragrant and translucent.

- Add the lean ground turkey or chicken to the pot and cook until browned, breaking it apart with a spoon as it cooks.
- Pour in the low-sodium chicken or vegetable broth, water, and diced tomatoes (including their juice). Stir well.
- Add the chopped broccoli, cauliflower, spinach or kale, and bell peppers to the pot. Season with dried thyme, dried rosemary, salt, and pepper. Mix everything together.
- Cover the pot and let the soup simmer for about 15-20 minutes, or until the vegetables are tender.
- If you'd like to add extra protein and fiber, you can stir in the cooked and drained kidney beans or chickpeas at this stage. Simmer for an additional 5 minutes.
- Taste and adjust the seasoning as needed.
- Serve the protein soup hot, garnished with fresh parsley if desired.

31

Quinoa and Black Bean Salad

This Quinoa and Black Bean Salad is not only diabetic-friendly but also packed with protein, fiber, and a variety of nutrients. It's a satisfying and nutritious option for a vegan meal.

```
Ingredients:
For the Salad:
1 cup quinoa, rinsed
2 cups water
1 (15-ounce) can black beans, drained and rinsed
1 cup cherry tomatoes, halved
1 cup cucumber, diced
1/2 cup red onion, finely chopped
1/4 cup fresh cilantro, chopped
1/4 cup fresh lime juice
Salt and pepper to taste
For the Dressing:
3 tablespoons olive oil
1 tablespoon balsamic vinegar
1 teaspoon Dijon mustard
1 teaspoon maple syrup (or a sugar substitute)
1 clove garlic, minced
1/2 teaspoon ground cumin
Salt and pepper to taste
```

Instructions:

- In a medium saucepan, combine the rinsed quinoa and water. Bring to a boil, then reduce heat, cover, and simmer for about 15 minutes, or until the quinoa is cooked and the liquid is absorbed. Remove from heat and let it cool.
- In a large salad bowl, combine the cooked and cooled quinoa, black beans, cherry tomatoes, cucumber, red onion, and fresh cilantro.
- In a small bowl, whisk together all the dressing ingredients: olive oil, balsamic vinegar, Dijon mustard, maple syrup (or sugar substitute), minced garlic, ground cumin, salt, and pepper.
- Pour the dressing over the salad and toss well to combine, ensuring all ingredients are coated.
- Drizzle the fresh lime juice over the salad and gently mix it in.
- Taste and adjust the seasoning, adding more salt, pepper, or lime juice as needed.
- Chill the salad in the refrigerator for at least 30 minutes before serving to allow the flavors to meld.

32

The Slim Fry

Ingredients:
For the Stir-Fry Sauce:
2 tablespoons low-sodium soy sauce
2 tablespoons rice vinegar
1 teaspoon sesame oil (use sparingly)
1 teaspoon cornstarch (or a diabetes-friendly thickener)
1 teaspoon minced fresh ginger
1 clove garlic, minced
1-2 teaspoons of a sugar substitute (like Stevia) (optional, for sweetness)

For the Stir-Fry:
2 boneless, skinless chicken breasts, cut into thin strips
2 cups mixed vegetables (e.g., bell peppers, broccoli, carrots, snap peas)
1 tablespoon vegetable oil (or a heart-healthy oil like olive oil)
1/2 onion, thinly sliced
2 cups cooked of cauliflower rice (as a low-carb alternative)
Sesame seeds and sliced green onions for garnish (optional)

Instructions:

Stir-Fry Sauce:

- In a small bowl, whisk together the low-sodium soy sauce, rice vinegar, sesame oil, cornstarch, minced ginger, minced garlic, and sugar substitute (if using). Set aside.

Stir-Fry:

- Heat the vegetable oil in a large skillet or wok over medium-high heat.
- Add the thinly sliced chicken strips to the hot skillet and stir-fry for 3-4 minutes or until cooked through and no longer pink in the center. Remove the cooked chicken from the skillet and set it aside.
- In the same skillet, add the sliced onion and mixed vegetables. Stir-fry for about 3-4 minutes until they start to become tender but are still crisp.
- Return the cooked chicken to the skillet and pour the stir-fry sauce over the chicken and vegetables.
- Continue to cook and stir for another 2-3 minutes, or until the sauce has thickened and everything is well coated.
- Serve the stir-fry over cooked brown rice or cauliflower rice for a lower-carb option.
- Garnish with sesame seeds and sliced green onions if desired.

33

Lem-O-salmon

```
Ingredients:
4 salmon fillets (about 6 ounces each)
2 lemons, juiced and zested
2 cloves garlic, minced
2 tablespoons fresh parsley, chopped
1 tablespoon fresh dill, chopped (or 1 teaspoon dried dill)
1 tablespoon olive oil
Salt and black pepper to taste
Lemon slices for garnish (optional)
```

Instructions:

- In a small bowl, whisk together the lemon juice, lemon zest, minced garlic, chopped parsley, chopped dill, olive oil, salt, and black pepper to create the marinade.
- Place the salmon fillets in a shallow dish or a large resealable plastic bag. Pour the marinade over the salmon, making sure each fillet is well-coated. Seal the bag or cover the dish and refrigerate for at least 30 minutes to allow the flavors to meld.
- Preheat your grill or oven to medium-high heat (about 400°F or 200°C).
- If grilling, lightly oil the grill grates to prevent sticking. If baking, line a

baking sheet with parchment paper or lightly grease it.

- Remove the salmon fillets from the marinade and place them on the grill or baking sheet. Discard the marinade.
- Grill the salmon for about 4-5 minutes per side or bake in the oven for 12-15 minutes, or until the salmon flakes easily with a fork and has a slightly crispy exterior.
- If desired, garnish with lemon slices before serving.

34

Mash It, Lose It

Purple Cauliflower is not only visually appealing but also a nutritious alternative to traditional mashed potatoes. Here's a simple recipe to make mashed purple cauliflower:

```
Ingredients:
1 head of purple cauliflower
2 cloves of garlic, minced
2 tablespoons olive oil
Salt and pepper to taste
2 tablespoons grated Parmesan cheese (optional for added flavor)
```

Instructions:

- Wash and chop the purple cauliflower into florets, removing any tough stems.
- Steam or boil the cauliflower until it's very tender, usually about 8-10 minutes.
- While the cauliflower is cooking, heat the olive oil in a pan over medium heat. Add the minced garlic and sauté for a minute or two until fragrant. Be careful not to brown the garlic; it should remain golden.

- Drain the cooked cauliflower and place it in a food processor or blender.
- Add the sautéed garlic, olive oil, salt, and pepper to the cauliflower.
- Blend until you achieve a smooth and creamy consistency, similar to mashed potatoes.
- If desired, mix in grated Parmesan cheese for added flavor.
- Taste and adjust the seasonings if necessary.

Serve your mashed purple cauliflower hot as a delicious and colorful side dish.

35

Apple Of My Eye

If you're experiencing nausea due to Ozempic and are looking for a diabetic-friendly dessert that may help soothe your stomach, consider trying a simple recipe for cinnamon applesauce. Cinnamon is known for its potential digestive benefits and can be soothing for nausea. Here's how to make it:

```
Ingredients:
2 apples (peeled, cored, and sliced)
1/2 teaspoon ground cinnamon
1/4 teaspoon nutmeg (optional)
1/4 cup water
Sugar substitute (if needed for sweetness, but use sparingly or
consider natural options like stevia or erythritol)
```

Instructions:

- Place the sliced apples, ground cinnamon, nutmeg (if using), and water in a saucepan.
- Cook over medium heat, stirring occasionally, until the apples become soft and start to break down. This usually takes about 10-15 minutes.
- If you'd like to sweeten the applesauce, add a small amount of a sugar substitute while it's still warm. Taste and adjust for sweetness.
- Let the applesauce cool, and then refrigerate it until you're ready to enjoy.

This homemade cinnamon applesauce is gentle on the stomach and provides some natural sweetness without spiking blood sugar levels. It's essential to keep portion sizes in check and monitor your blood sugar as needed. If nausea persists or worsens, consult with a healthcare professional for appropriate guidance and treatment.

36

Hot Choc-O

This diabetic-friendly hot chocolate is lower in sugar and carbohydrates compared to traditional hot chocolate. Be sure to choose a sugar substitute that works well for you and doesn't cause blood sugar spikes.

```
Ingredients :
1 cup unsweetened almond milk (or another low-sugar milk
alternative)
2 tablespoons unsweetened cocoa powder
1-2 tablespoons sugar substitute (such as stevia, erythritol, or
monk fruit), adjust to taste
1/4 teaspoon vanilla extract (optional for flavor)
A pinch of salt (optional)
Whipped cream or a small dollop of sugar-free whipped topping
(optional)
```

Instructions:

- In a saucepan, whisk together the unsweetened almond milk and unsweetened cocoa powder over medium heat.
- Heat the mixture while whisking until it's hot but not boiling.
- Add your sugar substitute of choice to the hot chocolate and stir until it's

fully dissolved. Adjust the sweetness to your liking.

· If you want to add extra flavor, stir in vanilla extract and a pinch of salt (if desired).

· Pour your hot chocolate into a mug.

· If you like, top it with a small dollop of sugar-free whipped cream or a sugar-free whipped topping.

37

O-pen Reservation

When dining out at restaurants while taking Ozempic, it's essential to make healthy food choices that help you maintain stable blood sugar levels. Here are some tips and suggestions for ordering at restaurants:

Opt for lean protein sources like grilled chicken, fish, lean cuts of beef or pork, tofu, or legumes. Avoid deep-fried or breaded options. If the restaurant offers whole-grain options, choose them over refined grains. For example, order brown rice, whole-grain pasta, or whole-grain bread when available. Sweet potatoes are always a better choice.

Request extra vegetables with your meal or choose dishes that are rich in vegetables. They provide fiber and nutrients without causing significant blood sugar spikes.

Watch Portion Sizes: Be mindful of portion sizes. Many restaurant servings are larger than necessary. Consider sharing a dish with a dining companion or requesting a half portion. Minimize your intake of high-carb dishes like pasta, pizza, white rice, and large quantities of bread.

Ask for sauces, dressings, and condiments on the side so that you can control the amount used. Avoid creamy or sugary sauces, and opt for vinaigrettes or low-sugar options. Choose water, unsweetened iced tea, tea, or water instead of sugary beverages.

Don't hesitate to ask your server about dietary accommodations or substitutions. Many restaurants are willing to accommodate special dietary needs. If you want dessert, consider sharing it with others at your table, or opt for a small fruit-based dessert.

Some restaurants provide nutritional information for their menu items. Review this information if available to make informed choices. If possible, review the restaurant's menu online before going out. This can help you make healthier choices in advance.

f you choose to have alcoholic beverages, do so in moderation, and be aware of the impact on your blood sugar levels.

Pay attention to your hunger and fullness cues. Stop eating when you're satisfied, even if there's food left on your plate.

Remember that individual dietary needs can vary, so it's crucial to consult with your healthcare provider or a registered dietitian for personalized guidance on managing your diabetes and making food choices that align with your treatment plan while taking Ozempic.

38

Ozempic-Friendly Snacks

Here are a few Ozempic-friendly snack ideas that are tasty, low in calories, easy to digest, and suitable for managing blood sugar levels:

Greek Yogurt Parfait:

Combine plain Greek yogurt with fresh berries (e.g., strawberries, blueberries, raspberries). Optionally, add a sprinkle of chopped nuts (e.g., almonds, walnuts) for extra crunch and healthy fats. Drizzle with a touch of honey or use a sugar substitute for sweetness.

Hummus and Veggies:

Serve fresh-cut vegetables like carrots, cucumbers, and bell peppers with a side of hummus for dipping. Veggies provide fiber, while hummus adds protein and flavor.

Mixed Nuts:

A small handful of unsalted mixed nuts (e.g., almonds, walnuts, pistachios) can be a satisfying and nutritious snack. Nuts provide healthy fats and protein to help keep you full.

Cottage Cheese with Fruit:

Top low-fat cottage cheese with diced fruit like pineapple, peaches, or mixed berries. Cottage cheese is a good source of protein, and the fruit adds natural sweetness.

Hard-Boiled Eggs:

Hard-boiled eggs are rich in protein and healthy fats. Sprinkle a little salt and pepper or your favorite seasoning for flavor.

Veggie Chips:

Make your own veggie chips by baking thinly sliced zucchini, sweet potatoes, or kale with a drizzle of olive oil. These provide a crunchy snack with fewer carbs than traditional potato chips.

Avocado Slices:

Enjoy avocado slices seasoned with a pinch of salt and pepper. The healthy fats in avocados help keep you satisfied.

Cucumber Roll-Ups:

Spread cream cheese or hummus on cucumber slices and roll them up. Add a dash of your favorite seasoning for extra flavor.

Roasted Chickpeas:

Toss chickpeas with olive oil and your choice of seasonings, then roast until crunchy. They provide fiber and protein in a convenient snack form.

Remember to monitor portion sizes and choose snacks that align with your dietary needs and preferences.

VI

Ozempic Real-Life Patient Experiences

39

John's Weight Loss Journey

John is a 52-year-old man with type 2 diabetes who has struggled to control his blood sugar levels and manage his weight. His healthcare provider prescribes Ozempic as part of his diabetes management plan. Over several months, John follows a balanced diet, increases his physical activity, and takes Ozempic as prescribed. He experiences gradual weight loss, improved blood sugar control, and increased energy levels. John's healthcare provider regularly monitors his progress and adjusts his treatment plan as needed.

40

Linda's Post-Pregnancy Diabetes Management

Linda, a 32-year-old mother, had always struggled with her weight, but after giving birth to her second child, she found it increasingly challenging to shed the extra pounds. She was also diagnosed with type 2 diabetes during her pregnancy, which further complicated her weight loss goals.

Linda's doctor suggested Wegovy as a potential solution to help her not only lose weight but also manage her diabetes more effectively. She was hesitant about taking medication while breastfeeding. The safety of Wegovy or Ozempic while breastfeeding is still up in the air. Although it is suspected that these drugs will not pass into breast milk and therefore not be absorbed by a breastfed infant, this hasn't definitively been proven

Linda continued to breastfeed for six months and lost some of her pregnancy weight. After this time, she stopped breastfeeding and moved her baby to formula.

At this point, Linda began her Wegovy journey, and within a few weeks, she started to notice significant changes. Her appetite decreased, and she felt full faster than before, making it easier to make healthier food choices. Linda also found that her blood sugar levels were stabilizing, reducing her dependence on insulin.

As Linda continued with Wegovy, the pounds began to melt away. She was overjoyed with the progress she was making and felt more energetic and confident as a mother of two. Linda combined the medication with regular exercise and a balanced diet, making it a holistic approach to her post-pregnancy weight loss.

Over time, Linda successfully reached her weight loss goals, shedding the pregnancy weight and more. She not only regained her pre-pregnancy figure but also improved her overall health.

41

Samantha's Journey to Overcoming Her Fear of Needles with Ozempic

Samantha's Journey to Overcoming Her Fear of Needles with Ozempic

Samantha, a 42-year-old mother of two, was excited to start her Ozempic treatment. She had struggled with obesity and type 2 diabetes for years, and her doctor recommended Ozempic as a potential solution to help her lose weight and manage her blood sugar levels.

However, Samantha had a deep-seated fear of needles that she had carried with her since childhood. The thought of self-injecting Ozempic was causing her significant anxiety. She knew the potential benefits of the medication, but her fear was holding her back.

Determined to face her fear and improve her health, Samantha sought the guidance of a nurse who specialized in teaching patients how to self-inject medications. The nurse provided Samantha with step-by-step instructions, offered emotional support, and allowed Samantha to practice with a placebo injection pen until she felt more confident.

Over time, Samantha's fear of needles began to diminish, and she was able to self-inject Ozempic with relative ease. It wasn't an overnight transformation, but Samantha's determination to overcome her fear and improve her health ultimately paid off.

As Samantha continued her Ozempic treatment, she started to see positive changes in her weight and blood sugar levels. Her story highlights the importance of seeking support and guidance when faced with challenges related to self-injecting medications, as well as the potential for personal growth and health improvement through determination and perseverance.

42

Mike's Long-Term Diabetes Management

Mike is a 68-year-old man who has been living with type 2 diabetes for several years. Despite previous medications, his blood sugar levels have not been well controlled, and he has concerns about weight gain. His healthcare provider prescribes Ozempic to address both issues. Mike follows a personalized diabetes management plan that includes Ozempic, dietary adjustments, and regular exercise. With this combination, he experiences improved blood sugar control and weight maintenance.

43

Tom's Transformation with Ozempic

Tom, a 55-year-old man, had struggled with his weight and multiple health issues for years. He was diagnosed with type 2 diabetes, high cholesterol, hypertension, and edema. His daily routine involved taking a handful of medications to manage these conditions, but despite his efforts, his health continued to deteriorate.

Tom's doctor recommended that he explore additional options to address his weight, as obesity was a significant contributing factor to his health problems. After discussing various treatment possibilities, they decided to give Ozempic a try.

Tom started on Ozempic while continuing his other medications. He was initially skeptical, given his previous unsuccessful attempts at weight loss. However, as the weeks went by, he began to notice significant changes. The pounds started to melt away, and his energy levels increased.

As the weight came off, Tom's blood sugar levels began to stabilize, and he experienced a notable improvement in his cholesterol numbers. His hypertension became easier to manage, and his edema lessened. Tom's doctor was pleased with his progress and began to reduce the dosages of some of his other medications.

With Ozempic's help, Tom managed to shed a substantial amount of weight, which had a cascading positive effect on his overall health. He continued to work closely with his healthcare team to monitor his progress and adjust his medications as needed. Tom's story serves as a testament to the potential transformative impact of Ozempic for individuals managing multiple health conditions alongside obesity.

44

Lisa And Her Poor Blood Sugar Control

Lisa is a 45-year-old woman who was diagnosed with type 2 diabetes five years ago. She has struggled to control her blood sugar levels despite taking multiple oral medications. Her A1c levels have consistently been above 8%, indicating poor glucose control. Lisa's healthcare provider decides to add Ozempic to her treatment plan to improve her blood sugar control. Lisa is already following a healthy diet and exercising regularly. She starts with a lower dose of Ozempic and gradually increases it over several weeks to minimize potential side effects.

Over the next few months, Lisa experiences significant improvements in her blood sugar levels. Her A1c drops to 6.5%, which is within the target range. She also notices a gradual reduction in her weight, improved energy levels, and fewer spikes in her blood sugar after meals. Lisa continues to work closely with her healthcare team to maintain her progress.

45

Randy Likes Carbohydrates

Randy is a 55-year-old man with a history of type 2 diabetes for over a decade. He has been managing his diabetes with a combination of oral medications and insulin injections. Despite his efforts, his blood sugar levels remain unstable, and he has gained weight over the years.

Randy's healthcare provider recommends transitioning him from insulin injections to Ozempic. They start by reducing his insulin dosage while initiating Ozempic therapy. Randy also receives education on adjusting his carbohydrate intake and monitoring his blood sugar closely during the transition.

With the guidance of his healthcare team, Randy successfully transitions to Ozempic and discontinues insulin injections. He notices a gradual decrease in his weight and improved blood sugar stability. Randy also experiences fewer episodes of hypoglycemia (low blood sugar), which were a concern with insulin therapy. His healthcare provider continues to monitor his progress and makes adjustments to his treatment plan as needed.

46

Harold's Weight Loss Journey with Ozempic and Pancreatitis

Harold, a 45-year-old accountant, had struggled with obesity and type 2 diabetes for most of his adult life. After years of unsuccessful attempts to lose weight through diet and exercise, his doctor recommended trying Ozempic to help manage his blood sugar levels and promote weight loss.

Harold was hopeful and excited to start Ozempic, as he had heard about its potential benefits. However, just a few weeks into the treatment, he began experiencing severe abdominal pain, nausea, and vomiting. He started having lightly colored and loose bowel movements. Concerned about these symptoms, Harold contacted his doctor. The doctor told him to stop the Ozempic immediately and ordered an ultrasound and blood work which confirmed the diagnosis of pancreatitis.

Pancreatitis is a rare but known side effect associated with some GLP-1 medications, including Ozempic. Harold was advised to stay off Ozempic and other GLP-1 medications. He required hospitalization for treatment of his pancreatitis. It was a challenging and painful experience for him.

Although Harold's journey with Ozempic was cut short due to this serious side effect, he continued working with his healthcare team to find alternative ways to manage his diabetes and obesity. His story serves as a reminder that while GLP-1 medications can be effective for many individuals, they are not without risks, and it's crucial to monitor for potential side effects and consult with healthcare professionals regularly.

47

Dylan The Heavy Diabetic

Dylan has had type 2 diabetes for many years and has struggled with obesity throughout his life. He's been on insulin therapy for several years to manage his blood sugar levels. Recently, Dylan's doctor introduced Ozempic to his treatment plan to help with both blood sugar control and weight management. Dylan's doctor adds Ozempic to his existing insulin regimen. As a result, he notices improved blood sugar control, reduced insulin requirements, and gradual weight loss. This helps Dylan feel more energetic and motivated to continue his diabetes management efforts. He also appreciates the convenience of a once-weekly injection, which is more manageable than multiple daily insulin injections.

48

Olivia's Journey: Shaping Up for the Big Day

Meet Olivia, a 30-year-old bride-to-be who had her dream wedding coming up in just six months. She had always wanted to look and feel her best on her special day, but there was one obstacle: she needed to shed about 15 pounds to fit perfectly into her dream wedding dress.

Olivia had heard about Wegovy from a friend who had successfully lost weight with it, so she decided to give it a try. She visited her healthcare provider, discussed her goals, and started on Wegovy as part of a comprehensive weight loss plan.

The journey wasn't always easy. Olivia had to make some changes to her diet and exercise routine, but Wegovy made it more manageable by reducing her appetite and helping her make healthier food choices. She also found herself feeling more motivated to stick to her plan, knowing that her wedding day was just around the corner.

As the months passed, Olivia's hard work and Wegovy's assistance paid off. She reached her goal of losing those 10 pounds, and her wedding dress fit like a dream. Olivia walked down the aisle with confidence and radiance, feeling beautiful and healthy on her big day.

Olivia's story demonstrates how Wegovy can be a helpful tool for individuals looking to achieve specific weight loss goals, even in a relatively short period. It's essential to remember that successful weight loss often requires a combination of medication, diet, exercise, and determination, as was the case for Olivia.

49

Trish's Remarkable Transformation with Ozempic

Trish, a vibrant 53-year-old, had always been a poster child for healthy living. However, as time passed and menopause approached, her tried-and-true habits seemed less effective. The COVID-19 pandemic made things worse, with her admitting that "the weight just kept piling on." Before her doctor prescribed Ozempic, she had managed to shed around 20 pounds (9 kilograms). But the results with Ozempic were truly life-altering. Trish lost a staggering 47 pounds (21 kilograms).

While she does experience some side effects like fatigue and occasional dizziness, she emphasizes that the benefits far outweigh any discomfort. For Trish, Ozempic has been nothing short of miraculous in overcoming the hurdles of traditional weight loss methods.

50

Renise's Ozempic Journey: Battling "Ozempic Face" to Regain Confidence

Renise, a 58-year-old retired nurse, had struggled with obesity for years. Many of her family members had diabetes and she was told she was at significant risk for that, having had high blood sugars during her pregnancies earlier in her life. Her doctor recommended Ozempic as a potential solution to help her lose weight and better manage her blood sugar. Excited about the prospects, Renise began her Ozempic journey with optimism.

However, as she continued with her Ozempic injections, she noticed a side effect that would later be coined as "Ozempic face" by some users. Renise's face appeared slightly swollen, especially around her cheeks and jawline. She also experienced mild puffiness around her eyes. Concerned about this unexpected side effect, Renise turned to online forums and support groups for advice.

Renise discovered that "Ozempic face" was a relatively common but usually temporary side effect experienced by some users. While it was challenging to deal with the change in her facial appearance, Renise decided to press on with her Ozempic treatment, focusing on the overall health benefits it was providing. She also found that some people sought out cosmetic specialists if they lost too much weight in their faces when taking Ozempic.

As weeks passed, Renise noticed her weight dropping steadily, and her blood sugar levels were better controlled. She also found that the facial puffiness gradually diminished over time, as her body adjusted to the medication. She saw no significant changes in the structure or shape of her face besides looking thinner to her friends and family. Her confidence began to grow as she saw positive changes in her health.

Renise's story illustrates the determination to overcome side effects and the importance of patience and perseverance in the journey towards better health. While "Ozempic face" was an initial hurdle, it didn't deter Karen from reaping the long-term benefits of Ozempic in her weight loss and diabetes management journey.

51

Ben's Wegovy Success Story

Ben's journey with Wegovy, a chemically identical Semaglutide injection to Ozempic designed for obesity and weight management, has been nothing short of inspiring. Like many others, Ben faced weight-related health issues, but his determination led him to try Wegovy. With the help of this medication, Ben has lost a significant amount of weight. He emphasizes that it's not just about shedding pounds but also transforming his relationship with food and exercise. To help with this, Ben has used a personal trainer to assist him to keep active. Ben mentions that he no longer craves unhealthy snacks and feels full faster. While he acknowledges having some side effects like nausea, he considers them a small price to pay for the positive changes in her life. Wegovy has given Ben renewed confidence and motivation to maintain a healthier lifestyle.

52

Tamar's Struggle with Ozempic

Tamar, a 45-year-old woman, had been battling her weight and mild type 2 diabetes for several years. She had tried numerous diets and exercise routines without much success. Frustrated with her lack of progress and concerned about her health, she turned to Ozempic as a potential solution.

Tamar started on a lower dose of Ozempic and diligently followed her doctor's recommendations. She hoped that this medication would finally help her shed the excess weight that had been a constant burden. However, as the weeks went by, Tamar saw no significant changes in her weight.

Determined to make it work, Tamar and her doctor decided to increase her Ozempic dosage gradually, eventually reaching the highest recommended dose. Despite her commitment, Tamar's weight remained stubbornly unchanged. She experienced some of the medication's side effects, including nausea and reduced appetite, but the desired weight loss eluded her.

Tamar's journey with Ozempic was a challenging one. She felt frustrated and disheartened, especially after investing so much time and effort into the treatment. Her healthcare team continued to monitor her progress and explored other options to address her weight and diabetes management.

While Tamar's story illustrates that Ozempic may not work the same way for everyone, it also underscores the importance of personalized healthcare and ongoing support in managing obesity and diabetes. Despite her initial setbacks, Tamar remained determined to improve her health and explore alternative approaches to achieve her weight loss goals.

53

Anonymous User's Journey with Wegovy

An individual who prefers to remain anonymous shared their experience with Wegovy, . Like many others, they had faced challenges with obesity for years, trying various diets and exercise routines without lasting success. After consulting with their healthcare provider, they decided to give Wegovy a try. The results were astonishing, as they lost a significant amount of weight. They reported experiencing some side effects like nausea and a decreased appetite for food. Despite these challenges, the weight loss and improved health outcomes were well worth it, and they felt more confident and energized in their daily life.

54

Jessica's Weight Loss Journey with Ozempic and Nausea

Jessica, a 42-year-old mother of two, had been battling weight gain and type 2 diabetes for several years. Her healthcare provider recommended trying Ozempic to help manage her blood sugar levels and support her weight loss goals. Jessica was excited about the potential benefits but was concerned about potential side effects, particularly nausea, as she had a history of motion sickness.

After starting Ozempic, Jessica did experience some nausea, especially during the first few weeks of treatment. It was challenging for her to eat her regular meals, and she often had to eat smaller portions to avoid discomfort. Despite these side effects, Jessica was determined to continue with the medication because she noticed positive changes in her blood sugar levels. Over time, the nausea gradually subsided, and Jessica adapted her diet to accommodate the medication.

In just a few months, Jessica lost over 20 pounds and saw significant improvements in her overall health. Her diabetes management became more manageable, and she had more energy to spend with her family. Jessica's story demonstrates that while nausea can be a common side effect when starting medications like Ozempic, it often improves with time, and the potential benefits of weight loss and better health can outweigh the initial discomfort.

55

Emma's Transformation with Ozempic: A Journey to Self-Confidence

Emma, a 38-year-old schoolteacher, had battled with weight issues for most of her adult life. She often felt self-conscious and struggled with her body image, which took a toll on her self-esteem and overall well-being. Despite numerous attempts at different diets and exercise regimens, significant weight loss had always seemed just out of reach.

When her doctor recommended Ozempic as part of her insulin-resistant management plan, Linda was initially skeptical but decided to give it a try. Over the course of several months, she experienced remarkable changes in her body. The pounds began to melt away, and her blood sugar levels stabilized.

However, what surprised Emma the most was how her perception of her body began to shift. As the weight came off, she started feeling more confident and comfortable in her own skin. Emma noticed that she was no longer overly critical of her appearance, and she began to embrace the changes in her body as signs of progress and health.

Emma's journey with Ozempic not only improved her physical health but also had a profound impact on her mental and emotional well-being. She learned to appreciate her body for its resilience and the progress she had made on her path to better health. Her story is a testament to how medications like Ozempic can do more than just aid in weight loss; they can also empower individuals to develop a more positive body image and regain their self-confidence.

56

Michelle's Ozempic Journey: Conquering Weight Loss, Confronting Constipation

Michelle, a 65-year-old woman with a borderline elevated Hemoglobin A1C, embarked on her weight loss journey with Ozempic, hoping to shed those extra pounds that had been bothering her for years. She had tried various diets and exercise plans in the past, but her struggles with weight loss seemed never-ending.

When Michelle's doctor suggested Ozempic as an option, she was eager to give it a try. She started the medication and immediately noticed a decrease in her appetite, which was a welcomed change. She began making healthier food choices and incorporated regular exercise into her routine.

However, Michelle encountered an unexpected challenge along the way: severe constipation. While Ozempic was helping her achieve her weight loss goals, it was also causing discomfort and digestive issues. Michelle tried increasing her fiber intake, drinking more water, and using over-the-counter remedies, but the constipation persisted.

She decided to consult her doctor about the issue. She was referred to a gastroenterologist who performed a colonoscopy. The results were all normal. In consultation with the specialist, her doctor adjusted her medication dosage and explored additional strategies to manage the side effects. This change helped alleviate some of the constipation symptoms, but Michelle still had to be mindful of her diet and hydration.

She began to read about severe constipation in people taking Ozempic. As a result, she was very nervous about continuing. However further discussion with her doctors confirmed that most of the reports of people with constipation were patients with existing diabetic gastroparesis before starting Ozempic.

Michelle never had constipation before starting the medication. Despite this setback, Michelle remained committed to her weight loss journey and continued Ozempic at a lower dose. With the support of her healthcare team, she successfully lost weight and improved her overall health, normalizing her hemoglobin A1C. Her experience highlights the importance of open communication with healthcare providers to address and manage potential side effects while working towards weight loss goals.

57

Kevin's Struggle to Access Ozempic: A Journey of Determination

Kevin, a 55-year-old man, had been living with type 2 diabetes for several years. His doctor recommended Ozempic as part of his diabetes management plan, emphasizing its potential to help him control his blood sugar levels and lose weight. Excited about the prospects of improved health, Kevin was eager to start the treatment.

However, when Kevin went to his local pharmacy to fill his prescription for Ozempic, he was taken aback by the high cost of the medication. Even with his insurance, the copay for Ozempic was prohibitively expensive, putting it out of reach for his budget as a retiree living on a fixed income.

Determined not to give up on his health, Kevin embarked on a journey to find a solution. He contacted his insurance company and explored various assistance programs offered by the manufacturer of Ozempic. It took time and effort, but eventually, Kevin was able to secure financial assistance that made the medication affordable for him.

As Kevin began his Ozempic treatment, he experienced significant improvements in his blood sugar control and started shedding excess weight. His perseverance paid off, and he realized that while the financial hurdles were daunting, there were resources available to help individuals access the medication they needed.

Kevin's story serves as a reminder that obtaining and affording medications like Ozempic can be challenging, but with determination and the right support, it's possible to overcome these obstacles and prioritize one's health.

VII

Conclusion

58

Future Trends in Diabetic and Obesity Treatment

Future trends in diabetic drug development are expected to focus on enhancing the efficacy, safety, and convenience of treatments for diabetes. As our understanding of the genetic and molecular factors contributing to diabetes grows, there will be a greater emphasis on personalized medicine. This involves tailoring treatments to an individual's specific genetic and metabolic profile to achieve optimal glycemic control and minimize side effects.

Advances in continuous glucose monitoring (CGM) technology and closed-loop insulin delivery systems (artificial pancreas) will continue to improve diabetes management. These systems aim to provide real-time glucose monitoring and automated insulin delivery, reducing the burden of diabetes management for patients.

While GLP-1 receptor agonists like Ozempic are currently administered by injection, research is ongoing to develop oral formulations of these drugs. This could significantly enhance convenience and patient adherence.

Sodium-glucose cotransporter-2 (SGLT-2) inhibitors have also gained popularity due to their ability to lower blood sugar and reduce cardiovascular risk. Future research will focus on refining these medications and understanding their long-term effects. Combination therapies that incorporate multiple mechanisms of action in a single medication will become more common. These combinations can improve glycemic control, reduce side effects, and simplify treatment regimens.

Biologic drugs, such as monoclonal antibodies, are being explored for their potential to target specific pathways involved in diabetes and related conditions. These therapies may offer novel treatment options with fewer side effects. Gene therapy approaches are being investigated to address the underlying genetic causes of certain types of diabetes. These therapies have the potential to provide long-term benefits by modifying the genes responsible for insulin production or regulation.

Nutritional interventions tailored to an individual's metabolic profile are gaining attention. Precision nutrition aims to optimize diet plans for better glycemic control and overall health. **Artificial intelligence and machine learning** algorithms are being used to analyze large datasets of patient information, helping identify patterns, predict disease progression, and optimize treatment plans.

The use of telemedicine and remote monitoring technologies will continue to grow, enabling healthcare providers to closely track and manage patients' diabetes remotely. Beyond treatment, there will be a greater focus on diabetes *prevention* strategies, including lifestyle interventions, early detection, and interventions to delay or prevent the onset of type 2 diabetes. Healthcare systems are increasingly moving toward patient-centered care models, where individuals with diabetes have a more active role in their treatment decisions and management plans.

The future of diabetic drug development is likely to be marked by greater personalization, integration of technology, and a holistic approach to diabetes management that goes beyond medication to address the broader health and well-being of individuals with diabetes. These trends aim to improve outcomes and quality of life for those living with diabetes.

Mounjaro (Tirzepatide) is a novel medication that falls under the class of drugs known as dual glucose-dependent insulinotropic peptide (GIP) and glucagon-like peptide-1 (GLP-1) receptor agonists. It is primarily being used for the treatment of type 2 diabetes and is designed to improve blood sugar control and provide additional benefits related to body weight and cardiovascular health.

Tirzepatide activates both the GIP and GLP-1 receptors, which are involved in regulating blood sugar levels and appetite. By stimulating these receptors, Tirzepatide increases the release of insulin (which lowers blood sugar) and suppresses the release of glucagon (which raises blood sugar). It also promotes feelings of fullness, which helps with weight management. It is also administered as a subcutaneous injection, typically once a week.

One of the notable features of Tirzepatide is its potential for promoting weight loss. Clinical trials have demonstrated significant reductions in body weight in individuals with type 2 diabetes who took Tirzepatide. The weight loss effect is believed to result from the combination of reduced appetite and improved blood sugar control.

Tirzepatide has also shown potential cardiovascular benefits in clinical trials, including a reduction in the risk of major adverse cardiovascular events (MACE) such as heart attacks and strokes. Tirzepatide's dual action on both GIP and GLP-1 receptors sets it apart from many other GLP-1 receptor agonists. This dual action may contribute to its robust effects on blood sugar control, weight loss, and cardiovascular outcomes.

Novo Nordisk, the Danish company that developed Ozempic, is actively engaged in ongoing research and development of GLP-1 receptor agonists with potential improvements in terms of dosing frequency, efficacy, and side effect profiles. In fact, the vast and growing popularity of Ozempic has led to Novo Nordisk the biggest boost this year to Denmark's economy. Eli Lilly, a major pharmaceutical company, had its GLP-1 receptor agonist called Trulicity (dulaglutide) on the market. They continued to explore new compounds and formulations in this category. AstraZeneca has a GLP-1 receptor agonist called Bydureon (exenatide extended-release) and was involved in research on next-generation GLP-1-based therapies. Sanofi is developing GLP-1 receptor agonists, including Adlyxin (lixisenatide), and exploring new compounds in this class. Various other pharmaceutical companies, including smaller biotech firms, were also engaged in the development of GLP-1 receptor agonists and related medications.

To compare Ozempic to other GLP-1 receptor agonists, it's essential to consider various factors, including their efficacy, dosing frequency, side effects, and specific characteristics.

Trulicity is another long-acting GLP-1 receptor agonist, typically administered once a week. Ozempic and Trulicity have similar mechanisms of action, aiming to improve blood sugar control and promote weight loss.

Bydureon is administered once a week and is another option for patients seeking less frequent dosing. Ozempic and Bydureon both aim to lower blood sugar levels and may lead to weight loss.

Victoza is a daily GLP-1 receptor agonist, whereas Ozempic is administered weekly. Both drugs are used for blood sugar control and weight management. Victoza may be chosen when daily dosing is preferred, while Ozempic offers the convenience of weekly injections. Adlyxin is a GLP-1 receptor agonist, but it is also typically administered as a once-daily injection.

Rybelsus (Oral Semaglutide) is used for type 2 diabetes and is the oral version of semaglutide, whereas Ozempic is administered as a weekly subcutaneous injection.

Oral semaglutide is also used for the treatment of type 2 diabetes. It has less efficacy (effectiveness) than injected semaglutide for both weight loss and diabetic control. Oral semaglutide can also promote a sense of fullness, which may contribute to weight loss in some individuals.

Oral semaglutide is typically taken once daily, usually in the morning, with or without food. It is important to follow the dosing instructions provided by a healthcare provider or on the medication label. Clinical trials have demonstrated that oral semaglutide is effective in improving glycemic control in people with type 2 diabetes. It can lower hemoglobin A1c (HbA1c) levels, reduce fasting and post-meal blood sugar levels, and help with weight management. The availability of an oral GLP-1 receptor agonist provides an alternative for individuals who prefer not to use injectable medications.

It offers a convenient option for managing diabetes without the need for needles.Common side effects of oral semaglutide can include nausea, vomiting, diarrhea, and abdominal discomfort. These side effects often diminish over time as the body adjusts to the medication.

Oral semaglutide, like other GLP-1 receptor agonists, may have cardiovas-cular benefits and is generally considered safe for most people with type 2 diabetes. However, it is important for individuals to discuss their medical history and any other medications they are taking with their healthcare provider to ensure that oral semaglutide is an appropriate treatment option.

It's important to note that oral semaglutide is just one of several treatment options available for type 2 diabetes. The choice of medication should be individualized based on factors such as a person's medical history, preferences, and treatment goals. Healthcare providers can help patients make informed decisions about the most suitable treatment plan for their specific needs.

Oral bioavailability refers to the extent and rate at which a drug or substance is absorbed into the bloodstream when taken orally (by mouth). Peptides are molecules made up of amino acids and can have a wide range of functions in the body, including as hormones, enzymes, and signaling molecules. The oral bioavailability of peptides can be challenging due to their susceptibility to enzymatic degradation and poor absorption through the digestive system. Here are some key considerations regarding the oral bioavailability of peptides:

When peptides are ingested orally, they encounter digestive enzymes in the stomach and small intestine, such as proteases. These enzymes break down proteins and peptides into smaller fragments, potentially reducing the bioavailability of intact peptides. Peptides typically have poor permeability across the intestinal wall. The gastrointestinal tract is designed to absorb nutrients efficiently, but peptides may face challenges in crossing the intestinal barrier due to their size and charge.

1. Chemical Modifications: To enhance oral bioavailability, researchers have explored various chemical modifications to peptides. These modifi-cations can make peptides more resistant to enzymatic degradation and improve their transport across the intestinal lining.

2. Prodrug Approaches: Prodrugs are inactive forms of drugs that are designed to convert into the active drug in the body. Prodrug strategies have been employed to improve the oral bioavailability of certain peptides.

3. Nanoparticles and Delivery Systems: Nanoparticles and drug delivery systems, such as nanoparticles, liposomes, and micelles, can encapsulate peptides, protect them from enzymatic degradation, and enhance their absorption.

4. Peptide Mimetics: Peptide mimetics are synthetic compounds designed to mimic the function of natural peptides while offering better oral bioavailability and stability.

5. Clinical Applications: Some peptide-based drugs are administered orally, such as certain medications for inflammatory bowel diseases. However, the success of oral peptide drugs can vary widely depending on the specific peptide, the formulation, and the disease being treated.

6. Ongoing Research: Ongoing research continues to explore innovative strategies to improve the oral bioavailability of peptides, as they hold promise for a wide range of therapeutic applications, including diabetes, metabolic disorders, and various diseases of the gastrointestinal tract.

It's important to note that while some peptides are successfully administered orally, the oral delivery of peptides remains a complex and evolving field. The development of effective oral peptide drugs often involves overcoming challenges related to stability, absorption, and enzymatic degradation in the digestive system. Each peptide and drug candidate may require a tailored approach to maximize its oral bioavailability.

When considering the choice between different GLP-1 receptor agonists, healthcare providers take into account individual patient needs, treatment goals, lifestyle factors, dosing preferences, and potential side effects. While these medications share a common class, they may have unique characteristics that make one more suitable than another for a particular patient.

There are scenarios where thin people might be prescribed Ozempic. While obesity is a common risk factor for type 2 diabetes, not all individuals with this condition are overweight or obese. Some people with a normal or low body weight can develop type 2 diabetes due to factors like genetics, insulin resistance, or lifestyle.

In some cases, healthcare providers may consider off-label use of Ozempic for specific medical conditions or weight management needs that fall outside the FDA-approved indications. Off-label use should be discussed thoroughly between the patient and the healthcare provider, taking into consideration potential benefits and risks.

Research is ongoing to explore the use of GLP-1 receptor agonists like semaglutide in various populations, including thin individuals, for conditions beyond diabetes and obesity. Clinical trials may investigate the effects of Ozempic in different patient groups to determine its safety and efficacy.

It's important to note that the decision to prescribe Ozempic or any medication is made by a qualified healthcare provider after a comprehensive evaluation of the patient's medical history, current health status, and treatment goals. The appropriateness of Ozempic for thin individuals would be determined on a case-by-case basis.

Additionally, the use of Ozempic, like any medication, should be accompanied by regular medical supervision and monitoring to ensure safety and effectiveness. Patients should consult with their healthcare provider to discuss their specific health needs and treatment options.

59

Mounjaro and Zepbound

Mounjaro, known generically as tirzepatide, is a groundbreaking medication that has recently garnered attention also for its potential in weight management. Initially developed and approved for the treatment of type 2 diabetes, Mounjaro's ability to significantly influence weight loss has sparked a new wave of interest and research

Mounjaro was first introduced as a treatment for type 2 diabetes, owing to its unique mechanism of action. It functions both as a glucose-dependent insulinotropic polypeptide (GIP) and glucagon-like peptide-1 (GLP-1) receptor agonist (through which Ozempic works). The dual action of Mounjaro helps regulate blood sugar levels by enhancing insulin secretion and suppressing glucagon release, but its effects on weight loss have become a focal point of recent studies. Because of the additional mechanism of action, Mounjaro has shown even greater weight loss in some patients than Ozempic or Semaglutide.

Dual GIP and GLP-1 receptor agonists work by mimicking the actions of both GIP and GLP-1. This means that they can stimulate insulin release from the pancreas in response to elevated blood sugar levels (glucose-dependent insulinotropic effect) and reduce the secretion of glucagon (which raises blood sugar levels) while also reducing appetite and promoting a feeling of fullness. By targeting both GIP and GLP-1 receptors, these medications provide a more comprehensive approach to blood sugar control. They help lower blood sugar levels by enhancing insulin secretion when it's needed (e.g., after a meal) and by reducing the production of glucose by the liver.

Clinical trials have shown that Mounjaro not only improves glycemic control but also leads to substantial weight loss in individuals with type 2 diabetes. Its weight-reducing effects are believed to stem from its action on appetite centers in the brain, leading to reduced food intake and increased feelings of fullness.

Based on the compelling evidence from clinical trials, Mounjaro has been sought for approval as a treatment for obesity or weight management in non-diabetic individuals. This new indication would mark a significant shift in the landscape of weight management therapies, offering a novel mechanism of action compared to existing treatments.

Most recently, the Food and Drug Administration has authorized tirzepatide as an agent only for weight loss. The pharmaceutical company that makes tirzepatide has released this new form as Zepbound. This is analgous to the release of Wegovy as the weight losing version of Semaglutide.

Mounjaro's potential for weight loss opens up new avenues for treating obesity. It can be prescribed for individuals struggling with weight issues, offering a new hope for effective management.

While Mounjaro has shown promising results, it is crucial to consider its safety profile. Like any medication, it comes with potential side effects, and its long-term effects on weight and overall health are still under investigation. Like Ozempic your doctor will need to weigh its benefits against potential risks, especially in non-diabetic patients.

Amongst the interesting investigational studies of terzipatide is the SUR-PASS trial which evaluated tirzepatide in people with type 2 diabetes. In the SURPASS-3 trial, tirzepatide demonstrated significant reductions in major adverse cardiovascular events, including cardiovascular death, non-fatal myocardial infarction (heart attack), and non-fatal stroke, when compared to placebo. This suggests a potential cardiovascular benefit associated with tirzepatide. Also, tirzepatide has been associated with improvements in lipid profiles, including reductions in LDL cholesterol and triglycerides, which are factors that can influence cardiovascular risk.

Similar to Ozempic, Mounjaro can cause gastrointestinal symptoms, such as nausea, vomiting, diarrhea, and abdominal pain. These symptoms may occur when you start taking tirzepatide but often improve over time. Gallbladder problems have happened in some people who use Mounjaro, as well as inflammation of the pancreas.

Tirzepatide may increase the risk of low blood sugar (hypoglycemia), especially when used in combination with other diabetes medications that lower blood sugar. Symptoms of hypoglycemia can include shakiness, sweating, rapid heartbeat, dizziness, confusion, and in severe cases, loss of consciousness.

Mounjaro's emerging role as a weight loss treatment represents a significant advancement in the field of obesity management. Its dual action mechanism offers a unique approach, distinguishing it from other weight loss medications. As research continues and its usage expands, Mounjaro could potentially become a cornerstone in the fight against obesity, changing countless lives for the better.

60

Closing Thoughts

As we journey through the pages of "The Ozempic Diet," we traverse the fascinating pathway of Ozempic's discovery, its groundbreaking role in the landscape of weight loss medications, and the intricacies of nourishing oneself harmoniously while on this treatment. The anecdotes of individual patients, each with their unique challenges and triumphs, have added a human touch to this scientific expedition, reminding us of the profound impact these advancements have on everyday lives.

The future of weight loss medications is a vast, ever-evolving horizon. Ozempic is just one beacon in this expansive sky, but its luminescence has illuminated a path for many who have been seeking direction. As promising as it is, it's essential to remember that no medication is an island. The context in which it is consumed—the food we eat, the lifestyle choices we make, the awareness we have of potential side effects—determines its true efficacy.

The stories shared in this book, both of molecular innovation and human perseverance, underscore a singular truth: holistic well-being is achieved not just through a pill but through an integrated approach that respects both science and individuality. As you close this book, it is my hope that you're equipped with not just knowledge but also a renewed sense of hope and empowerment. The journey towards health is a personal one, filled with its unique challenges, but with the right tools and understanding, it's a journey filled with promise.

As we stand on the cusp of more medical innovations, let's also celebrate the age-old wisdom of listening to our bodies, making informed choices, and finding balance. Here's to a brighter, healthier future for all, with the magic of medicine and the power of informed choices walking hand in hand.

The journey through "The Ozempic Diet" has been both illuminating and transformative. We've ventured together from the foundational discovery of Ozempic to the promising horizons of weight loss medications. The stories of individual triumphs, challenges, and resilience have provided living testimony to the transformative potential of the right intervention, complemented by informed choices.

Yet, as with any medical odyssey, it's essential to remember that while Ozempic heralds a new dawn in weight management, it is not a magic bullet. The harmony between the medication and the body is significantly influenced by the foods we consume and the manner in which we eat. Nourishing oneself goes beyond mere caloric intake; it's about choosing foods that resonate with our metabolic symphony, optimizing the benefits of the medication, and minimizing potential side effects.

The personal accounts interspersed throughout the book have underlined a fundamental truth: every individual's journey is unique. While Ozempic provides a common thread, the tapestry of each life, with its patterns of challenges, side effects, and successes, is singularly distinctive.

Looking to the future, the landscape of weight loss medications is vibrant and dynamic. Ozempic, pioneering as it is, represents just one star in a rapidly expanding universe. As research progresses and our understanding deepens, there will undoubtedly be newer interventions, refined guidelines, and more tales of transformation.

However, the core principle will remain unaltered: Medications offer tools, not solutions. The ultimate power lies in informed, conscious choices and a commitment to one's well-being. The pages of this book have aimed to empower you with knowledge, insights, and a holistic perspective. Armed with this, you are better positioned to navigate your health journey with confidence, discernment, and optimism.

The diagnosis of diabetes often comes with a mix of disbelief, fear, and a sense of helplessness. But it's crucial to understand that while diabetes is a chronic condition, it's also a manageable one. The power to live a full, vibrant life with diabetes lies, to a significant extent, in the hands of the patient. Reclaiming control begins with the acceptance of the diagnosis and a commitment to work collaboratively with healthcare professionals. With the right mindset, education, and actions, diabetes can become a manageable part of one's life, rather than an overwhelming force.

Building a strong relationship with your healthcare provider is paramount. While patients steer their health journey, doctors serve as invaluable co-pilots, offering guidance, expertise, and support. Regular check-ups, open communication, and mutual trust form the bedrock of this relationship. Understand that your doctor's advice springs from a place of knowledge and a genuine desire to see you thrive.

Food plays a central role in diabetes management. But "eating right" doesn't mean adhering to a restrictive, joyless diet. It's about understanding how different foods affect your blood sugar and crafting a nourishing, tasty, and sustainable eating plan. Familiarize yourself with the glycemic index, learn the benefits of whole foods, and recognize the role of portion control. Remember, every meal is an opportunity to nourish your body.

Beyond food, several aspects of daily life influence diabetes control. Exercise, stress management, adequate sleep, and regular monitoring of blood sugar levels play crucial roles. By integrating healthy habits into daily routines and staying consistent, patients can greatly influence the course of their diabetic journey. It's not about radical changes, but consistent, mindful choices.

Medications can be invaluable allies in diabetes management. They can assist in maintaining target blood sugar levels, reducing complications, and improving quality of life. However, like all interventions, they come with their set of benefits and potential side effects. Being informed about your prescribed medications, understanding their action, and being vigilant about any adverse reactions is crucial. Medications are tools - their efficacy hinges on how judiciously they're used.

The overarching message is one of empowerment. While external resources like doctors, medications, and support groups are vital, the most potent force in diabetes management is the patient. Embrace your agency, educate yourself, seek support when needed, and remember: diabetes is a part of your journey, not its entirety. With the right approach, you can not only live with diabetes but thrive in spite of it.

As we close this chapter, remember that every end is a new beginning. May "The Ozempic Diet" serve as a steadfast companion in your quest for optimal health and inspire you to chart your path with wisdom and grace.

61

Appendices

- Wegovy™ is a **trademark of Novo Nordisk A/S.**
- Ozempic™ is a **trademark of Novo Nordisk A/S.**
- Mounjaro™ **is a trademark of Eli Lilly and Company**
- Zepbound™ **is a trademark of Eli Lilly and Company**
- Victoza™ **is a trademark of Novo Nordisk A/S.**
- Byetta™/Bydureon™ **is a trademark of Astra Zeneca.**
- Trulicity™ **is a trademark of Eli Lilly and Company**
- Saxenda™ is a **trademark of Novo Nordisk A/S.**
- Rybelsus™ is a **trademark of Novo Nordisk A/S.**

The future development of GLP-1 inhibitors holds significant potential to advance the treatment of diabetes, obesity, and related metabolic disorders. These advancements may lead to more effective, convenient, and personalized therapies that improve the lives of millions of individuals living with these conditions. Continued research, innovation, and collaboration between pharmaceutical companies, healthcare professionals, and researchers will be instrumental in shaping this future landscape.

Dual glucose-dependent insulinotropic polypeptide (GIP) and glucagon-like peptide-1 (GLP-1) receptor agonists are a class of medications developed for the treatment of type 2 diabetes and obesity. These drugs are designed to address both of these metabolic conditions by simultaneously targeting two key hormones involved in regulating blood sugar and metabolism: GIP and GLP-1.

Pharmaceutical companies continue to invest in research and development to create new GLP-1-based and new GIP-based therapies and improve existing ones. The field of these new drugs is dynamic, with ongoing efforts to enhance the effectiveness, convenience, and safety of these treatments for patients with type 2 diabetes, obesity, and other metabolic disorders. Several pharmaceutical companies are actively involved in the development and manufacturing of GLP-1 and GIP drugs and many of these agents are in late-phase clinical trials and will soon come to market, opening up a larger (and more competitive) fight in this extremely lucrative commercial healthcare space.

62

Studies and References

The studies detailed below offer a glimpse into some of the larger and more pivotal clinical trials concerning GLP-1 (Glucagon-Like Peptide-1) agents, yet it's crucial to recognize that this collection is far from exhaustive. The field of GLP-1 research is a dynamic and ever-evolving one, with ongoing investigations and breakthroughs constantly expanding our understanding of these important agents. These selected studies highlight the significant impact of GLP-1 receptor agonists on diabetes management, weight loss, and cardiovascular outcomes, but they are just a fraction of the broader body of research that continues to shape the future of metabolic medicine.

SUSTAIN 7: Head-to-head vs Trulicity (dulaglutide)[2]

Study design: 40-week, multinational, multicenter, randomized, open-label, 4-armed, pairwise, active-controlled, parallel-group trial to compare the efficacy and safety of Ozempic vs dulaglutide.

Patients: A total of 1201 adult patients with type 2 diabetes inadequately controlled on metformin were randomized to receive Ozempic 0.5 mg (n=301), Ozempic 1 mg (n=300), dulaglutide 0.75 mg (n=299), or dulaglutide 1.5 mg (n=299) once weekly.

Primary endpoint: Mean change in A1C from baseline at Week 40.

Secondary endpoints: Mean change in body weight from baseline at Week

40; proportion of patients achieving A1C <7% at Week 40.

SUSTAIN 4: Head-to-head vs Lantus (insulin glargine U-100)[1,5]

Study design: 30-week, randomized, open-label, active-controlled, parallel-group, multinational, multicenter trial to compare the efficacy and safety of Ozempic® vs insulin glargine U-100.

Patients: A total of 1089 insulin-naïve adult patients with type 2 diabetes inadequately controlled on metformin alone (48%) or in combination with a sulfonylurea (51%) were randomized to receive once-weekly Ozempic 0.5 mg (n=362), once-weekly Ozempic 1 mg (n=360), or once-daily insulin glargine U-100 (n=360). Patients assigned to insulin glargine had a baseline mean A1C of 8.1% and were started on a dose of 10 units once daily. Insulin glargine dose adjustments occurred throughout the trial period based on self-measured fasting plasma glucose before breakfast, targeting 71 to <100 mg/dL. In addition, investigators could titrate insulin glargine based on their discretion between study visits. Twenty-six percent of patients had been titrated to goal by the primary endpoint at Week 30, at which time the mean daily insulin dose was 29 units per day.

Primary endpoint: Mean change in A1C from baseline at Week 30.

Secondary endpoints: Mean change in body weight from baseline at Week 30; proportion of patients achieving A1C <7% at Week 30.

SUSTAIN 5: As an add-on to basal insulin vs placebo

Study design: 30-week, randomized, double-blind, placebo-controlled, parallel-group, multinational, multicenter trial to compare the efficacy and safety of Ozempic in combination with basal insulin vs volume-matched placebo in combination with basal insulin.

Patients: A total of 397 adult patients inadequately controlled on basal insulin with or without metformin were randomized to once-weekly Ozempic 0.5 mg (n=132), Ozempic 1 mg (n=131), or placebo (n=133). Randomization was stratified according to A1C at screening. Patients with A1C ≤8% at screening reduced the insulin dose by 20% at the start of the trial to reduce the risk of hypoglycemia.

Primary endpoint: Mean change in A1C from baseline at Week 30.

Secondary endpoints: Mean change in body weight from baseline at Week 30; proportion of patients achieving A1C <7% at Week 30; change in mean fasting plasma glucose (FPG) at Week 30.

Sustain FORTE: Ozempic 1 mg vs 2 mg

Study design: 40-week, randomized, active-controlled, parallel-group, double-blind, phase 3B efficacy and safety trial of Ozempic 2 mg vs Ozempic 1 mg in patients with type 2 diabetes in need of treatment intensification.

Patients: A total of 961 adult patients with inadequately controlled type 2 diabetes (A1C 8.0%-10.0%) on metformin with or without a sulfonylurea were randomized 1:1 to 2.0 mg (n=480) or 1.0 mg (n=481) of once-weekly Ozempic.

Primary endpoint: Mean change in A1C from baseline at Week 40.

Secondary endpoints: Mean change in body weight from baseline at Week 40; proportion of patients achieving change in body weight >5% or ≤10% at Week 40.

Weight regain and cardiometabolic effects after withdrawal of semaglutide: The STEP 1 trial extension

Aim To explore changes in body weight and cardiometabolic risk factors after treatment withdrawal in the STEP 1 trial extension.

Materials and Methods STEP 1 randomized 1961 adults with a body mass index ≥ 30 kg/m2 (or ≥ 27 kg/m2 with ≥1 weight-related co-morbidity) without diabetes to 68 weeks of once-weekly subcutaneous semaglutide 2.4 mg (including 16 weeks of dose escalation) or placebo, as an adjunct to lifestyle intervention. At week 68, treatments (including lifestyle intervention) were discontinued. An off-treatment extension assessed for a further year a representative subset of participants who had completed 68 weeks of treatment. This subset comprised all eligible participants from any site in Canada, Germany and the UK, and sites in the United States and Japan with the highest main phase recruitment. All analyses in the extension were exploratory.

Results Extension analyses included 327 participants. From week 0 to week 68, mean weight loss was 17.3% (SD: 9.3%) with semaglutide and 2.0% (SD: 6.1%) with placebo. Following treatment withdrawal, semaglutide and placebo participants regained 11.6 (SD: 7.7) and 1.9 (SD: 4.8) percentage points of lost weight, respectively, by week 120, resulting in net losses of 5.6% (SD: 8.9%) and 0.1% (SD: 5.8%), respectively, from week 0 to week 120. Cardiometabolic improvements seen from week 0 to week 68 with semaglutide reverted towards baseline at week 120 for most variables.

Conclusions One year after withdrawal of once-weekly subcutaneous semaglutide 2.4 mg and lifestyle intervention, participants regained two-thirds of their prior weight loss, with similar changes in cardiometabolic variables. Findings confirm the chronicity of obesity and suggest ongoing treatment is required to maintain improvements in weight and health.

Semaglutide 2·4 mg once a week in adults with overweight or obesity, and type 2 diabetes (STEP 2): a randomised, double-blind, double-dummy, placebo-controlled, phase 3 trial

Background This trial assessed the efficacy and safety of the GLP-1 analogue once a week subcutaneous semaglutide 2·4 mg versus semaglutide 1·0 mg (the dose approved for diabetes treatment) and placebo for weight management in adults with overweight or obesity, and type 2 diabetes.

Methods This double-blind, double-dummy, phase 3, superiority study enrolled adults with a body-mass index of at least 27 kg/m2 and glycated haemoglobin 7–10% (53–86 mmol/mol) who had been diagnosed with type 2 diabetes at least 180 days before screening. Patients were recruited from 149 outpatient clinics in 12 countries across Europe, North America, South America, the Middle East, South Africa, and Asia. Patients were randomly allocated (1:1:1) via an interactive web-response system and stratified by background glucose-lowering medication and glycated haemoglobin, to subcutaneous injection of semaglutide 2·4 mg, or semaglutide 1·0 mg, or visually matching placebo, once a week for 68 weeks, plus a lifestyle intervention. Patients, investigators, and those assessing outcomes were masked to group assignment. Coprimary endpoints were percentage change in bodyweight and achievement of weight reduction of at least 5% at 68 weeks for semaglutide 2·4 mg versus placebo, assessed by intention to treat. Safety was assessed in all patients who received at least one dose of study drug.

Results From June 4 to Nov 14, 2018, 1595 patients were screened, of whom 1210 were randomly assigned to semaglutide 2·4 mg (n=404), semaglutide 1·0 mg (n=403), or placebo (n=403) and included in the intention-to-treat analysis. Estimated change in mean bodyweight from baseline to week 68 was −9·6% (SE 0·4) with semaglutide 2·4 mg vs −3·4% (0·4) with placebo. Estimated treatment difference for semaglutide 2·4 mg versus placebo was −6·2 percentage points (95% CI −7·3 to −5·2; p<0·0001). At week 68, more patients on semaglutide 2·4 mg than on placebo achieved weight reductions of at least 5% (267 [68·8%] of 388 vs 107 [28·5%] of 376; odds ratio 4·88, 95% CI 3·58 to 6·64; p<0·0001). Adverse events were more frequent with semaglutide 2·4 mg (in 353 [87·6%] of 403 patients) and 1·0 mg (329 [81·8%] of 402) than with placebo (309 [76·9%] of 402). Gastrointestinal adverse events, which were mostly mild to moderate, were reported in 256 (63·5%) of 403 patients with semaglutide 2·4 mg, 231 (57·5%) of 402 with semaglutide 1·0 mg, and 138 (34·3%) of 402 with placebo.

Conclusions In adults with overweight or obesity, and type 2 diabetes, semaglutide 2·4 mg once a week achieved a superior and clinically meaningful decrease in bodyweight compared with placebo.

Effect of Subcutaneous Semaglutide vs Placebo as an Adjunct to Intensive Behavioral Therapy on Body Weight in Adults With Overweight or Obesity: The STEP 3 Randomized Clinical Trial

Background: To compare the effects of once-weekly subcutaneous semaglutide, 2.4 mg vs placebo for weight management as an adjunct to intensive behavioral therapy with initial low-calorie diet in adults with overweight or obesity.

Methods Randomized, double-blind, parallel-group, 68-week, phase 3a study (STEP 3) conducted at 41 sites in the US from August 2018 to April 2020 in adults without diabetes (N = 611) and with either overweight (body mass index ≥27) plus at least 1 comorbidity or obesity (body mass index ≥30) Participants were randomized (2:1) to semaglutide, 2.4 mg (n = 407) or placebo (n = 204), both combined with a low-calorie diet for the first 8 weeks and intensive behavioral therapy (ie, 30 counseling visits) during 68 weeks.

Findings In this randomized clinical trial that included 611 adults with overweight or obesity, 68 weeks' treatment with once-weekly subcutaneous semaglutide vs placebo, combined with intensive behavioral therapy (and a low-calorie diet for the initial 8 weeks), resulted in reductions in body weight of 16.0% vs 5.7%, respectively; the difference was statistically significant.

Results Of 611 randomized participants (495 women [81.0%], mean age 46 years [SD, 13], body weight 105.8 kg [SD, 22.9], and body mass index 38.0 [SD, 6.7]), 567 (92.8%) completed the trial, and 505 (82.7%) were receiving treatment at trial end. At week 68, the estimated mean body weight change from baseline was −16.0% for semaglutide vs −5.7% for placebo (difference, −10.3 percentage points [95% CI, −12.0 to -8.6]; $P < .001$). More participants treated with semaglutide vs placebo lost at least 5% of baseline body weight (86.6% vs 47.6%, respectively; $P < .001$). A higher proportion of participants in the semaglutide vs placebo group achieved weight losses of at least 10% or 15% (75.3% vs 27.0% and 55.8% vs 13.2%, respectively; $P < .001$). Gastrointestinal adverse events were more frequent with semaglutide (82.8%) vs placebo (63.2%). Treatment was discontinued owing to these events in 3.4% of semaglutide participants vs 0% of placebo participants.

Conclusions Among adults with overweight or obesity, once-weekly subcutaneous semaglutide compared with placebo, used as an adjunct to intensive behavioral therapy and initial low-calorie diet, resulted in significantly greater weight loss during 68 weeks. Further research is needed to assess the durability of these findings.

Effect of Continued Weekly Subcutaneous Semaglutide vs Placebo on Weight Loss Maintenance in Adults With Overweight or ObesityThe STEP 4

Randomized Clinical Trial

Question What effect does continued treatment with 2.4 mg of subcutaneous semaglutide have on the maintenance of body weight loss in adults with overweight or obesity without diabetes?

Findings In this randomized clinical trial of adults with overweight or obesity, 803 participants completed a 20-week run-in of weekly treatment with subcutaneous semaglutide, 2.4 mg, with a mean weight loss of 10.6%, and were randomized to continued treatment with subcutaneous semaglutide vs placebo for an additional 48 weeks. At the end of this time, mean weight change was −7.9% vs +6.9%, respectively, a difference that was statistically significant.

Objective To compare continued once-weekly treatment with subcutaneous semaglutide, 2.4 mg, with switch to placebo for weight maintenance (both with lifestyle intervention) in adults with overweight or obesity after a 20-week run-in with subcutaneous semaglutide titrated to 2.4 mg weekly.

Design, Setting, and Participants Randomized, double-blind, 68-week phase 3a withdrawal study conducted at 73 sites in 10 countries from June 2018 to March 2020 in adults with body mass index of at least 30 (or ≥27 with ≥1 weight-related comorbidity) and without diabetes.

Interventions A total of 902 participants received once-weekly subcutaneous semaglutide during run-in. After 20 weeks (16 weeks of dose escalation; 4 weeks of maintenance dose), 803 participants (89.0%) who reached the 2.4-mg/wk semaglutide maintenance dose were randomized (2:1) to 48 weeks of continued subcutaneous semaglutide (n = 535) or switched to placebo (n = 268), plus lifestyle intervention in both groups.

Main Outcomes and Measures The primary end point was percent change in body weight from week 20 to week 68; confirmatory secondary end points were changes in waist circumference, systolic blood pressure, and physical functioning (assessed using the Short Form 36 Version 2 Health Survey, Acute Version [SF-36]).

Results Among 803 study participants who completed the 20-week run-in period (with a mean weight loss of 10.6%) and were randomized (mean age, 46 [SD, 12] years; 634 [79%] women; mean body weight, 107.2 kg [SD,

22.7 kg]), 787 participants (98.0%) completed the trial and 741 (92.3%) completed treatment. With continued semaglutide, mean body weight change from week 20 to week 68 was -7.9% vs +6.9% with the switch to placebo (difference, -14.8 [95% CI, -16.0 to -13.5] percentage points; $P < .001$). Waist circumference (-9.7 cm [95% CI, -10.9 to -8.5 cm]), systolic blood pressure (-3.9 mm Hg [95% CI, -5.8 to -2.0 mm Hg]), and SF-36 physical functioning score (2.5 [95% CI, 1.6-3.3]) also improved with continued subcutaneous semaglutide vs placebo (all $P < .001$). Gastrointestinal events were reported in 41.9% of participants who continued subcutaneous semaglutide vs 26.1% with placebo; similar proportions discontinued treatment because of adverse events with continued semaglutide (2.4%) and placebo (2.2%).

Conclusions Among adults with overweight or obesity who completed a 20-week run-in period with subcutaneous semaglutide, 2.4 mg once weekly, maintaining treatment with semaglutide compared with switching to placebo resulted in continued weight loss over the following 48 weeks.

Two-year effect of semaglutide 2.4 mg on control of eating in adults with overweight/obesity: STEP 5

Objective This study evaluated the effect of once-weekly semaglutide 2.4 mg on 2-year control of eating.

Methods In STEP 5, adults with overweight/obesity were randomized 1:1 to semaglutide 2.4 mg or placebo, plus lifestyle modification, for 104 weeks. A 19-item Control of Eating Questionnaire was administered at weeks 0, 20, 52, and 104 in a subgroup of participants. P values were not controlled for multiplicity.

Results In participants completing the Control of Eating Questionnaire (semaglutide, n = 88; placebo, n = 86), mean body weight changes were -14.8% (semaglutide) and -2.4% (placebo). Scores significantly improved with semaglutide versus placebo for Craving Control and Craving for Savory domains at weeks 20, 52, and 104 (p < 0.01); for Positive Mood and Craving for Sweet domains at weeks 20 and 52 (p < 0.05); and for hunger and fullness at week 20 (p < 0.001). Improvements in craving domain scores were positively correlated with reductions in body weight from baseline to week

104 with semaglutide. At 104 weeks, scores for desire to eat salty and spicy food, cravings for dairy and starchy foods, difficulty in resisting cravings, and control of eating were significantly reduced with semaglutide versus placebo (all $p < 0.05$).

Conclusions In adults with overweight/obesity, semaglutide 2.4 mg improved short- and longer-term control of eating associated with substantial weight loss.

Made in the USA
Las Vegas, NV
10 May 2024

89765812R00125